Rose Mary Romano

DIABETIC DIET AFTER 50

A Comprehensive Guide and Cookbook For Managing Type 2 Diabetes
With 180 Tasty, Easy-To-Make Low-Carb and Low-Sugar Recipes,
Practical Lifestyle Modifications and a 30-Day Meal Plan for Optimal Well-Being

Unlock Your Exclusive Extras Here!

In appreciation for your choice of this book, **I am happy to offer you 3 Additional Extra Contents** that can be downloaded in just a few steps by scanning the QR code.

Your feedback matters!

D1716040

Table of Contents

INTRODUCTION

When people reach the age of 50 and beyond, it becomes extremely important for them to take care of their health, especially those who are coping with type 2 diabetes. When it comes to efficiently managing blood sugar levels and encouraging general well-being, a specialized approach to eating becomes absolutely necessary. The diabetic diet for those over the age of 50 emphasizes the importance of creating a balance between engaging in healthy eating habits and making decisions about their lives.

Foods that are high in nutrients should be prioritized. The incorporation of a wide range of colorful vegetables, lean proteins, whole grains, and healthy fats facilitates the regulation of blood sugar levels and contributes to the maintenance of general health. It is just as crucial to limit portions because it helps with weight management and avoids spikes in blood glucose that are not essential from occurring.

People who are above the age of 50 and are following to a diabetic diet may find that monitoring their consumption of carbs becomes increasingly important. A significant factor in preventing sudden shifts in blood sugar levels is the selection of complex carbohydrates that have a low glycemic index. Incorporating foods that are high in fiber, such as fruits, vegetables, and whole grains, into one's diet helps to maintain energy levels throughout time and improves one's ability to control their blood sugar levels.

Timing meals consistently is an important component in the management of type 2 diabetes. Maintaining regular eating habits is beneficial for maintaining stable blood sugar levels during the day. Moreover, maintaining an adequate level of hydration is not only vital for overall health but also can assist in the regulation of appetite.

Individualized dietary plans, which are developed in collaboration with medical specialists, play a significant role in the process of adapting nutritional strategies to the specific requirements and preferences of each individual. Dietary efforts are complemented by regular physical activity, which contributes to increased insulin sensitivity and overall health.

In order to accomplish optimal blood sugar management and to maintain a healthy lifestyle, a diabetic diet for individuals over the age of 50 who have type 2 diabetes comprises an integrated approach. This strategy combines mindful food choices, portion control, regular meal timing, and individualized tactics.

DIABETES AFTER 50

Overview of Type 2 Diabetes

The inability of the body to make efficient use of insulin is the root cause of type 2 diabetes, which is a metabolic condition that encompasses the entire population. It is an essential hormone that generally regulates blood sugar levels, which in turn makes it easier for cells to absorb glucose for the purpose of obtaining energy. The manifestation of type 2 diabetes occurs when the body either makes insufficient insulin or confronts tolerance to the actions of insulin within cells, which results in hyperglycemia. This is in contrast to type 1 diabetes, which occurs when insulin production is insufficient.

The onset of type 2 diabetes is typically slow, and there is a discernible increase in the prevalence of the condition as persons age, particularly once they reach the age of 50. This increased risk in the population that is getting older is caused by a number of different reasons, including age-related changes in metabolism, decreased physical activity, and the possibility of accumulating extra weight over the course of one's lifetime.

In addition, the intricacy of type 2 diabetes is further highlighted by the complicated interaction between genetic predisposition, lifestyle choices, and environmental factors. There is a considerable increase in the chance of having this ailment due to lifestyle factors such as sedentary routines, inadequate food habits, and obesity.

Despite the fact that symptoms such as more thirst, regular urination, unexplained weight loss, and exhaustion are classic signs of type 2 diabetes, there are some people who may not exhibit any symptoms at all. This highlights the importance of routine health check-ups, particularly for those who are over the age of 50.

Modifications to one's lifestyle that are thorough are required in order to eradicate type 2 diabetes successfully. The adoption of a healthy weight, the participation in regular physical exercise, and the maintenance of a balanced diet are all essential components of management measures. In certain circumstances, medical practitioners may suggest the use of insulin therapy or medicine to help in the regulation of blood sugar levels.

As the proportion of people aged 65 and older who have type 2 diabetes continues to rise, the importance of taking preventative measures and detecting the disease at an early stage becomes more and more pressing. Regular monitoring of blood sugar levels, the adoption of a lifestyle that is health conscious, and timely medical intervention are all factors that assist cumulatively in the successful management and overall well-being of diabetes.

Risk Factors

There are several factors that affect the likelihood of acquiring diabetes after the age of 50, and each of these factors has a unique impact on the intricate nature of this metabolic disorder. People's physiological dynamics change with age, and these changes may make them more susceptible to diabetes, especially type 2.

- **Age:** An elevated risk of diabetes is closely associated with the natural aging process. The body's metabolism may slow down and insulin resistance may worsen after turning 50, which can have a major impact on the development of diabetes.

- **Genetics and Family History:** It is impossible to ignore one's genetic legacy. An affecting sign that suggests a genetic predisposition to diabetes is a family history of the disease. People over 50 may be on a possibly higher-risk trajectory if their parents or siblings have struggled with diabetes.

- **Lifestyle Choices:** Our daily decisions, particularly those pertaining to nutrition and exercise, have a significant impact on how well we feel about our health. As people get older, a propensity for sedentary behavior combined with unhealthy eating habits may solidify, creating an environment that is favorable to weight gain and insulin resistance. In the 50+ age range, maintaining an active lifestyle becomes essential to preventing diabetes.

- **Obesity:** After the age of 50, being overweight - especially in the abdomen - becomes a substantial risk factor for type 2 diabetes. The tendency to acquire weight during this period of life can be further exacerbated by hormonal changes and a possible loss of muscular mass.

- **Medical History:** People over 50 who have underlying medical issues like high blood pressure, PCOS, or cardiovascular disease are more likely to develop diabetes. This emphasizes the significance of managing one's health holistically.

- **Ethnicity:** Diabetes is more common in some ethnic groups than others. People of African American, Hispanic, Native American, and Asian American descent may experience a higher risk after the age of fifty, which highlights the importance of specific preventive actions.

- **Gestational Diabetes:** Women who have gestational diabetes during pregnancy have a higher chance of type 2 diabetes in later life, particularly after turning 50.

- **Hormonal Changes:** The complex network of factors impacting diabetes risk in the post-50 demographic includes menopause in women as well as age-related hormonal variations in both genders that might affect insulin sensitivity.

- **Sleep Disorders:** Poor sleep quality and sleep apnea, which may become more common as people age, have been related to a higher risk of diabetes. Sleep changes may have an impact on an individual's vulnerability to diabetes after the age of fifty.

IMPORTANCE OF DIET IN CONTROLLING DIABETES

Role of Diet

It is essential to observe a diet that is well-balanced in order to effectively manage and prevent diabetes, especially type 2 diabetes. In addition to having a direct influence on blood sugar levels, weight, and overall health, it gives people the ability to make educated decisions that are beneficial to their health.

- **Balancing Macronutrients:** Carbohydrates, proteins, and fats are the three macronutrients that need to be carefully maintained in order to create a diet that is suitable for diabetics. Whole grains, legumes, and vegetables are examples of complex carbohydrates that have a low glycemic index. Consuming these types of carbohydrates can help prevent abrupt spikes in blood glucose levels. Consuming meals that are high in fiber in conjunction with carbohydrates helps to maintain a steady release of energy and improves glycemic monitoring. When it comes to satiety and overall health, the contribution of proteins derived from lean sources and healthy fats derived from nuts, seeds, avocados, and olive oil cannot be overstated.

- **Portion Control:** Managing portion sizes is essential due to the fact that it plays a significant role in both the management of calorie intake and the prevention of excessive consumption. Smaller, more well-balanced meals spread out throughout the day are more successful in regulating blood sugar levels than big meals that are eaten only occasionally. This helps with weight management, which is an essential component of diabetes prevention.

- **Emphasizing Whole Foods:** A diet that is suitable for people with diabetes should largely consist of foods that are whole and unprocessed. These foods should include items such as fruits, vegetables, whole grains, lean proteins, and healthy fats. The use of these reduces the amount of added sugars, refined carbohydrates, and harmful fats that are consumed, while simultaneously providing critical nutrients, fiber, and antioxidants.

- **Dietary Fiber:** Fiber is an essential component in the management of diabetes conditions. Because it slows down the rate at which sugar is absorbed, soluble fiber, which can be discovered in fruits, vegetables, legumes, and whole grains, helps to prevent sudden rises in blood glucose. The feeling of fullness that is promoted by insoluble fiber is beneficial to the health of the digestive system and helps with weight management.

- **Strategic Meal Timing:** Maintaining an ongoing meal timing schedule helps to regulate blood sugar levels by synchronizing the consumption of food with the natural insulin production of the body. Consuming food at consistent intervals throughout the day allows for the prevention of excessive changes in blood glucose levels, which in turn promotes steady levels of energy.

- **Limiting Added Sugars and Processed Foods:** It is essential to reduce the amount of processed foods and added sugars you consume in order to effectively manage diabetes. The use of these goods is associated with an increase in calorie intake, weight gain, and fluctuations in blood sugar levels. The adoption of a healthier eating pattern can be facilitated by examining food labels in order to discover hidden sugars and selecting alternatives that are whole and unprocessed.

- **Individualized Approach:** Understanding the one-of-a-kind nature of dietary requirements is crucial. The formulation of individualized dietary programs that are suited to an individual's health goals, preferences, and cultural concerns can be accomplished through consultation with healthcare specialists, including registered dietitians.

- **Hydration:** Maintaining a sufficient amount of hydration is essential for a lifestyle that is diabetes-friendly. Water facilitates digestion, contributes to general health, and assists in maintaining healthy blood sugar levels. Hydration and management of blood sugar levels can be improved by choosing beverages that do not contain sugar, such as water or juice, rather than sugary drinks.

- **Regular Monitoring and Adaptation:** Keeping a close eye on your blood sugar levels and making adjustments to your diet on a consistent basis can give you with significant information. It makes it possible to make adjustments based on accurate information and make continuing treatment of diabetes easier, so ensuring a proactive approach to health.

Nutritional Management

When it comes to diabetes care, nutritional management is an essential component because it has an impact on blood sugar levels, overall health, and overall well-being. The following is a collection of useful recommendations for people who have diabetes on the management of sugars, carbohydrates, lipids, and other necessary nutrients.

- **Managing Sugars:** It is essential for people who have diabetes to exercise control over the amount of sugar they consume. The natural sugars that can be found in fruits as well as the added sugars that can be found in processed foods need to be taken into consideration. Choose fruits that are whole since they include critical minerals and fiber, both of which slow down the rate at which sugar is absorbed. Limit your consumption of sugary beverages, sweets, and snacks. The ability to read food labels is essential for locating sugars that are concealed in packaged goods. Take into consideration the use of natural alternatives such as stevia or monk fruit when sweetening foods or beverages. These alternatives have a limited impact on the levels of sugar in the blood.

- **Carbohydrate Management:** Because carbohydrates have a direct impact on blood sugar levels, careful management of carbohydrates is an essential component of diabetes treatment. Whole grains, legumes, and vegetables are examples of complex carbohydrates that have a low glycemic index. It is very important to prioritize the consumption of these types of carbohydrates. Because these carbohydrates are digested more slowly, they prevent spikes in blood glucose from occurring too quickly. The regulation of portions is of the utmost importance, and the distribution of carbohydrate consumption throughout the day in the form of smaller, more well-balanced meals is an efficient method for regulating blood sugar levels. It is possible to gain insight into an individual's tolerance levels by monitoring their blood sugar responses to various types of carbohydrates such as carbohydrates.

- **Understanding Fiber:** Diabetic management can benefit greatly from the use of dietary fiber. It adds to a feeling of fullness, helps maintain healthy digestive function, and helps maintain stable blood sugar levels. Foods that are high in fiber, such as fruits, vegetables, legumes, and whole grains, should be consumed. In particular, soluble fiber can be of assistance in the management of blood sugar levels by reducing the rate at which glucose is absorbed into the body. Instead than relying on supplements, people should think about getting their fiber from complete, unprocessed foods.

- **Healthy Fats:** It is essential to incorporate nutrient-dense fats into your diet if you want to feel satisfied and healthy overall. Nuts, olive oil, avocados, and fatty seafood like salmon are all good sources of unsaturated fats. Choose these foods whenever possible. It is important to limit your consumption of saturated and trans fats, which are frequently found in processed meals, fried foods, and certain oils. Due to the greater calorie content of fats, it is essential to monitor portion sizes of fats. This is because fats might have an effect on weight control, which is an important concern in diabetes care.

- **Protein Intake:** Protein has a crucial role in both the preservation of muscle mass and the promotion of overall health at the same time. Choose lean protein sources such as fish, chicken, lentils, and tofu instead of other options. If you want to avoid consuming an excessive amount of calories, pay attention to the portion sizes. The management of hunger and blood sugar levels during meals can be aided by the consumption of snacks that are high in protein.

- **Portion Control:** One of the most important principles related to diabetes management is controlling portion sizes. A number of factors contribute to good portion management, including the use of smaller plates, the measurement of food, and awareness of the suggested serving sizes. Not only does this technique assist in the regulation of blood sugar levels, but it also aids initiatives aimed at weight management.

- **Meal Timing and Consistency:** The establishment of a regular meal schedule is beneficial for the control of diabetes. Meal timing and regularity are also important considerations. In order to prevent irregular variations in blood sugar, it is important to maintain regular meal times and to prevent missing meals. A more steady energy level and better regulation of glucose levels can be achieved by distributing food consumption throughout the day in the form of well-balanced meals and snacks.

- **Hydration:** Proper hydration is frequently neglected, despite the fact that it is significant for both overall health and the control of diabetes. Water is the greatest option, and adequate hydration can be achieved by drinking it at regular intervals throughout the day. Sugary drinks, particularly fruit juices, should be consumed with caution because they can lead to an increase in the amount of sugar consumed.

- **Regular Monitoring:** When blood sugar levels are monitored often, it is possible to obtain valuable feedback regarding the influence of dietary choices taken. Keeping a meal diary and noting the responses of your blood sugar to the food helps uncover patterns and allows you to make modifications based on accurate information. When individuals visit healthcare specialists on a regular basis, particularly registered dietitians, they are able to receive individualized advice that is tailored to their specific health requirements.

- **Individualized Approach:** It is essential to acknowledge that different people have different nutritional requirements. Things that are successful for one individual might not be appropriate for an extra. It is helpful to consult with professionals in the healthcare field in order to build a personalized dietary plan that takes into account the preferences of the individual, the cultural influences, and the particular health goals.

The Right List of Ingredients

It is necessary for a diabetic diet to include a number of elements that has been carefully reviewed, particularly for people who are now over the age of 50. This list includes a wide variety of food categories in order to guarantee a well-balanced and nutrient-rich approach to the management of blood sugar levels and the promotion of general health. A breakdown of the categories is as follows:

Vegetables:

- Leafy greens (spinach, kale, collard greens)
- Non-starchy vegetables (broccoli, cauliflower, peppers)
- Root vegetables in moderation (sweet potatoes, carrots)

Fruits:

- Berries (blueberries, strawberries, raspberries)
- Apples and pears (in moderation, with the skin for added fiber)
- Citrus fruits (oranges, grapefruits)

Whole Grains:

- Quinoa
- Brown rice
- Oats
- Whole wheat products (bread, pasta)

Lean Proteins:

- Skinless poultry (chicken, turkey)
- Fish (salmon, trout, tuna)
- Lean cuts of beef or pork
- Tofu and tempeh for plant-based options

Legumes:

- Lentils
- Chickpeas
- Black beans
- Kidney beans

Healthy Fats:

- Avocado
- Nuts (almonds, walnuts)
- Seeds (flaxseeds, chia seeds)
- Olive oil for cooking and salad dressings

Dairy or Dairy Alternatives:

- Low-fat or fat-free yogurt
- Skim milk
- Unsweetened almond or soy milk

Non-Starchy Snack Options:

- Raw vegetables with hummus
- Handful of nuts
- Greek yogurt with berries
- Cheese slices or cubes (in moderation)

Herbs and Spices:

- Fresh herbs (parsley, cilantro, basil)
- Spices (cinnamon, turmeric, cumin) for flavor without added salt or sugar

Beverages:

- Water
- Herbal teas (unsweetened)
- Sparkling water with a splash of citrus for variety

Sweeteners (in moderation):

- Stevia
- Monk fruit
- Small amounts of honey or maple syrup

Portion-Controlled Treats (occasional):

- Dark chocolate (70% cocoa or higher)
- Sugar-free gelatin
- Small servings of dessert made with sugar substitutes

Low-Fat Dairy Options (in moderation):

- Cottage cheese
- Low-fat cheese

Condiments (used sparingly):

- Mustard
- Vinegar
- Salsa (without added sugars)

Whole Grain Snacks:

- Whole grain crackers
- Air-popped popcorn (unsalted)

Hydration:

- Water with lemon or cucumber
- Unsweetened herbal teas
- Infused water with mint or berries

PERSONALIZED MEAL PLANS

Meal Plans Overview

Personalised meal plans are an essential component in the successful management of diabetes. These plans provide an individualised approach to nutrition that is in accordance with the specific health requirements, preferences, and lifestyle alterations of the individual. These plans go past a one-size-fits-all approach, taking into account the specific elements of each individual's health profile, such as their age, weight, level of activity, and any preexisting medical issues. When it comes to the management of diabetes, individualized meal plans show a great deal of potential in terms of increasing blood sugar control and other aspects of overall health and wellness.

1. **Tailored Nutritional Approaches:** Tailored to the Individual Customized meal plans take into account the individual's nutritional needs, ensuring that an adequate balance of macronutrients—carbohydrates, proteins, and fats—is maintained. Managing carbohydrate consumption is especially important for people who have diabetes, and a tailored strategy takes into account the individual's tolerance to carbohydrates, which helps prevent rises in blood sugar levels.

2. **Blood Sugar Control:** Within the context of diabetes management, one of the key goals of individualized meal planning is to properly regulate blood sugar levels. The goal of these programs is to limit changes in blood glucose levels by deliberately splitting meals and snacks throughout the day, taking into consideration the glycemic index of foods, and implementing portion control. This will promote stability and reduce the risk of hyperglycemia.

3. **Weight Management:** A significant number of people who have diabetes may also be striving toward weight management or maintaining a healthy weight. In personalized meal plans, calorie requirements are taken into consideration, and an emphasis is placed on nutrient-dense meals that contribute to feelings of fullness and overall wellness. In light of the fact that being overweight can make insulin resistance worse, this individualized approach helps support weight-related goals, which is an essential component of diabetes therapy.

4. **Lifestyle Considerations:** In addition to the nutritional components, tailored meal plans take into account lifestyle characteristics such as the amount of physical activity, the job schedule, and the cultural preferences of the individual. This holistic approach acknowledges that in order to become sustainable, dietary modifications must be aligned with the daily routines and habits of an individual. This ensures that the prescribed meal plan will be adhered to over the long run.

5. **Cultural Sensitivity:** When developing a meal plan that is both functional and culturally sensitive, it is crucial to understand and appreciate the cultural background and dietary customs of the individual being planned for. This aspect helps to cultivate a sense of inclusiveness, which in turn makes the meal plan more practical and attuned to the individual's capabilities.

6. **Education and Empowerment:** Individuals who have diabetes are often provided with an educational component that is included in personalized meal plans. This enables them to make educated decisions regarding their food selections. The purpose of this education is to acquire practical skills in meal preparation and planning, as well as an understanding of the influence that various foods have on blood sugar levels, their interpretation, and the interpretation of food labels.

7. **Regular Monitoring and Adjustments:** The adaptability of personalized meal plans is a dynamic character trait that makes them unique. In order to make necessary adjustments to the meal plan, it is necessary to do regular monitoring of blood sugar levels and occasional check-ins with healthcare specialists, particularly registered dietitians. By doing this continuing assessment, the plan is guaranteed to continue to be in accordance with the individual's ever-changing health status and objectives.

8. **Collaborative Approach:** The process of developing individualized meal plans is a cooperative endeavor that involves both the individuals themselves and medical professionals such as certified dietitians. By fostering a sense of ownership over one's health, promoting active participation in the decision-making process, and supporting adherence to the meal plan, this collaborative method helps individuals feel ownership over their own health.

Tasty Recipes

BREAKFAST RECIPES

1. Vegetable Omelet with Spinach and Tomatoes

Preparation time: 10 minutes
Cooking time: 5 minutes
Servings: 1
Ingredients:

- 2 eggs
- 1/4 cup spinach, cut into small bits
- 1/4 cup tomatoes, cubed
- Salt and pepper as needed
- 1 tsp olive oil

Directions:

9. After the eggs have been whisked in the bowl, they ought to be flavored with salt and pepper before being served.
10. In a pan that does not stick, bring the olive oil to a temp. that is somewhere in the middle.
11. After adding cut into small bits spinach and cubed tomatoes to the pan, sauté the mixture for two to three minutes.
12. After the veggies have been topped with the whisked eggs, simmer them until they are set, raising the edges of the dish to allow the uncooked eggs to run below.
13. Following the completion of the cooking process, fold the omelet in half and place it on a platter.
14. Provide quickly.

Per serving: Calories: 280kcal; Fat: 20g; Carbs: 5g; Protein: 18g; Sugar: 3g

2. Veggie Breakfast Burrito with Whole Wheat Tortilla

Preparation time: 15 minutes
Cooking time: 10 minutes
Servings: 2
Ingredients:

- 2 whole wheat tortillas
- 4 eggs, scrambled
- 1/2 cup black beans, that is drained and washed
- 1/2 cup cubed bell peppers
- 1/4 cup cubed onions
- Salsa and avocado for topping

Directions:

1. Begin by sautéing cubed onions and bell peppers in your skillet until they have become more tender.
2. Include scrambled eggs and black beans, and continue to heat until the eggs are at the desired level of doneness.
3. Keep the tortillas made from whole wheat warm.
4. Split the egg mixture among the tortillas in a single layer.
5. Using a cut into small bits avocado and salsa, top the dish.
6. Then, present the burritos that you rolled out.

Per serving: Calories: 350kcal; Fat: 12g; Carbs: 40g; Protein: 18g; Sugar: 3g

3. Almond Butter & Banana Sandwich on Whole Grain Bread

Preparation time: 5 minutes
Cooking time: 0 minutes
Servings: 1
Ingredients:

- 2 slices whole grain bread
- 2 tbsps almond butter (unsweetened)
- 1 banana, cut

Directions:

1. Disperse almond butter so that it is evenly distributed on one side of every slice of bread.
2. Arrange banana slices on one slice of bread, and then finish with the other slice of bread, with the almond butter side facing down.
3. Create a sandwich by applying light pressure.
4. If it is necessary, cut it in half, and then use it.

Per serving: Calories: 380kcal; Fat: 18g; Carbs: 50g; Protein: 10g; Sugar: 15g

4. Whole Grain Toast with Smashed Avocado & Cherry Tomatoes

Preparation time: 10 minutes
Cooking time: 0 minutes
Servings: 1
Ingredients:

- 1 slice whole grain bread, toasted
- 1/2 ripe avocado, smashed
- 1/2 cup cherry tomatoes, divided
- Salt and pepper as needed
- Fresh cilantro or basil for garnish

Directions:

1. To begin, take the whole grain bread and toast it to your desire.
2. Distribute the mashed avocado in a spreadable manner across the toast.
3. Top with cherry tomatoes that have been split.
4. Include salt and pepper as needed, depending on the situation.
5. A garnish of fresh basil or cilantro is recommended.
6. Present instantly.

Per serving: Calories: 250kcal; Fat: 15g; Carbs: 25g; Protein: 5g; Sugar: 2g

5. Berry Smoothie Bowl with Chia Seeds

Preparation time: 10 minutes
Cooking time: 0 minutes
Servings: 1
Ingredients:

- 1 cup mixed berries (strawberries, blueberries, raspberries)
- 1/2 banana, frozen
- 1/2 cup unsweetened almond milk
- 1 tbsp chia seeds
- Toppings: cut almonds, shredded coconut

Directions:

1. Put the frozen banana, mixed berries, and almond milk into a mixer and mix

them together. Blend until it is completely smooth.

2. Put the smoothie into a bowl and set it aside.

3. Sprinkle some chia seeds on top.

4. If preferred, incorporate shredded coconut and uncut almonds into the mixture.

5. Use a spoon to scoop it up.

Per serving: Calories: 280kcal; Fat: 12g; Carbs: 35g; Protein: 8g; Sugar: 15g

6. *Turkey and Vegetable Breakfast Skillet*

Preparation time: 10 minutes
Cooking time: 15 minutes
Servings: 2
Ingredients:

- 1/2 lb ground turkey
- 1 bell pepper, cubed
- 1 zucchini, cubed
- 1 tsp olive oil
- 4 eggs
- Salt and pepper as needed
- Fresh parsley for garnish

Directions:

1. Bring the olive oil to a temp. that is in the middle of your skillet.

2. Include ground turkey, then wait until it has browned before serving.

3. Adding cut into small bits bell pepper and zucchini and continue to simmer until the vegetables are cooked.

4. Fourth, move the turkey and vegetables to the side of the skillet and put them away.

5. Crack the eggs into the skillet, flavor them with salt and pepper, and cook them according to your preferences.

6. Whisk the entire components together, and then top with cut into small bits fresh parsley.

7. Serve while still hot.

Per serving: Calories: 340kcal; Fat: 18g; Carbs: 10g; Protein: 30g; Sugar: 5g

7. *Cucumber and Tomato Breakfast Salad*

Preparation time: 10 minutes
Cooking time: 0 minutes
Servings: 2
Ingredients:

- 1 cucumber, cubed
- 1 cup cherry tomatoes, divided
- 1/4 cup red onion, finely cut into small bits
- 2 tbsps feta cheese, crumbled
- 1 tbsp olive oil
- 1 tbsp balsamic vinegar
- Salt and pepper as needed
- Fresh basil for garnish

Directions:

1. Put the cut into small bits cucumber, cherry tomatoes, red onion, and crumbled feta cheese in the bowl you have chosen.

2. In the small bowl you have, blend the balsamic vinegar and olive oil by whisking them together. Place on top of the salad, then toss to evenly distribute the dressing.

3. Include salt and pepper as needed, depending on the situation.

4. Top with some fresh basil for garnish.

5. This salad can be served as a cooling breakfast option.

Per serving: Calories: 160kcal; Fat: 12g; Carbs: 12g; Protein: 4g; Sugar: 6g

8. Broccoli and Cheese Egg Muffins

Preparation time: 15 minutes

Cooking time: 20 minutes

Servings: 4

Ingredients:

- 6 eggs
- 1 cup broccoli, finely cut into small bits
- 1/2 cup cheddar cheese, shredded
- Salt and pepper as needed
- Cooking spray

Directions:

1. Warm up your oven to 375 deg.F, and then spray a muffin tray with cooking spray to oil it.

2. Crack the eggs into your bowl and flavor them with salt and pepper before beating them.

3. Stir in the shredded cheddar cheese and the cut into small bits broccoli that you have prepared.

4. In a regular manner, pour the ingredients into the muffin tin that you have.

5. Bake the egg muffins for 20 minutes, or until they have reached the desired consistency and have a golden hue.

6. Before taking it from the tin, wait for it to cool down.

7. Serve at a warm temp.

Per serving: Calories: 180kcal; Fat: 12g; Carbs: 5g; Protein: 12g; Sugar: 2g

9. Apple Cinnamon Quinoa Muffins

Preparation time: 15 minutes

Cooking time: 25 minutes

Servings: 6

Ingredients:

- 1 cup cooked quinoa
- 1/2 cup applesauce (unsweetened)
- 1/4 cup almond flour
- 1/2 tsp cinnamon
- 1/4 tsp nutmeg
- 2 eggs
- 1/4 cup honey
- 1/2 tsp baking powder
- 1/4 tsp salt

Directions:

1. Warm up your oven to 350 deg.F. Next, line a muffin tin with paper liners.

2. Blend the cooked quinoa, applesauce, almond flour, nutmeg, cinnamon, eggs, honey, baking powder, and salt in a bowl.

3. Fill the muffin cups with the batter.

4. Bake until a toothpick immersed into the center comes out clean, around 25 minutes.

5. Allow it to cool before delivering.

Per serving: Calories: 180kcal; Fat: 6g; Carbs: 28g; Protein: 5g; Sugar: 12g

10. Smoked Salmon and Cream Cheese Bagel (Whole Wheat)

Preparation time: 5 minutes
Cooking time: 0 minutes
Servings: 1

Ingredients:

- 1 whole wheat bagel, cut and toasted
- 2 tbsps cream cheese (reduced-fat)
- 2 oz. smoked salmon
- Capers and fresh dill for garnish

Directions:

1. Evenly distribute the cream cheese over the toasted bagel halves.
2. Top with smoked salmon.
3. Include some fresh dill and capers as garnish.
4. Present instantly.

Per serving: Calories: 320kcal; Fat: 12g; Carbs: 40g; Protein: 18g; Sugar: 2g

11. Avocado and Egg Breakfast Bowl

Preparation time: 10 minutes
Cooking time: 5 minutes
Servings: 1

Ingredients:

- 1 ripe avocado, divided and pitted
- 2 eggs
- Salt and pepper as needed
- Fresh herbs (e.g., chives, parsley) for garnish

Directions:

1. Make a well for the egg by scooping a small amount of avocado flesh from either half of the avocado.

2. To avoid the avocados falling out of the baking dish, put them within the dish.
3. Break an egg into each half of the avocado.
4. Flavor with salt and pepper, according as needed specifications.
5. Bake the eggs in an oven that has been preheated to 375 deg.F for around 12 to 15 minutes, or until they are cooked to your satisfaction.
6. Afterwards, offer the dish with a garnish of fresh herbs.

Per serving: Calories: 330kcal; Fat: 25g; Carbs: 14g; Protein: 12g; Sugar: 1g

12. Quinoa Breakfast Porridge with Almonds

Preparation time: 5 minutes
Cooking time: 15 minutes
Servings: 2

Ingredients:

- 1/2 cup quinoa, washed
- 1 cup unsweetened almond milk
- 1/2 tsp vanilla extract
- 1/4 cup almonds, cut into small bits
- Fresh berries for topping (optional)

Directions:

1. Put the quinoa, almond milk, and vanilla essence into your pot and mix them together.
2. Bring to a boil, then decrease the temp. to a low setting, cover, and continue to simmer for 15 minutes, or until the quinoa is cooked and the mixture has thickened out.
3. Stir in the freshly cut into small bits almonds.

4. Split the mixture into bowls and, if desired, garnish with fresh berries.

Per serving: Calories: 300kcal; Fat: 12g; Carbs: 35g; Protein: 10g; Sugar: 2g

13. Cottage Cheese Pancakes with Berries

Preparation time: 10 minutes
Cooking time: 10 minutes
Servings: 2
Ingredients:

- 1 cup cottage cheese
- 2 eggs
- 1/2 cup whole wheat flour
- 1 tsp baking powder
- 1/2 tsp vanilla extract
- Mixed berries for topping

Directions:

1. Put the cottage cheese, eggs, ground whole wheat flour, baking powder, and vanilla extract in a mixer and beat until combined. Blend until it is completely smooth.
2. Bring the temp. of a non-stick skillet up to the middle.
3. The third step is to pour a quarter cup of batter for every pancake onto your griddle.
4. Cook until bubbles appear on the surface, then flip it over and keep cooking the other side until it reaches a golden brown color.
5. Perform the same steps with the leftover batter.
6. Place a mixture of berries on top of the pancakes.

Per serving: Calories: 300kcal; Fat: 8g; Carbs: 30g; Protein: 20g; Sugar: 6g

14. Spinach and Feta Frittata

Preparation time: 15 minutes
Cooking time: 15 minutes
Servings: 2
Ingredients:

- 4 eggs, beaten
- 1 cup fresh spinach, cut into small bits
- 1/4 cup feta cheese, crumbled
- 1/2 cup cherry tomatoes, divided
- Salt and pepper as needed
- 1 tsp olive oil

Directions:

1. Warm up the broiler in your oven.
2. Blend the beaten eggs, cut into small bits spinach, feta cheese, and cherry tomatoes in the basin you have designated for this purpose.
3. Include salt and pepper as needed (flavoring).
4. In an oven-safe skillet, bring the olive oil to a temp. that is in the middle.
5. Pour the egg mixture into the skillet, and then continue to cook it for 3 to 4 minutes, or until the edges become firm.
6. After that, move the skillet to the oven and continue to broil it for an extra three to 5 minutes, until the top is set and has a golden flavor.
7. Afterward, slice and then present.

Per serving: Calories: 280kcal; Fat: 20g; Carbs: 6g; Protein: 18g; Sugar: 3g

15. Sweet Potato Hash with Poached Eggs

Preparation time: 15 minutes
Cooking time: 20 minutes
Servings: 2
Ingredients:

- 2 medium sweet potatoes, skinned and grated
- 1 onion, finely cut into small bits
- 1 bell pepper, cubed
- 2 eggs (poached)
- 1 tbsp olive oil
- Salt and pepper as needed
- Fresh parsley for garnish

Directions:

1. Bring the olive oil to a temp. that is in the middle of your skillet.
2. Include cut into small bits onions and continue to sauté until they become transparent.
3. Include grated sweet potatoes and cubed bell pepper in the skillet containing the ingredients.
4. Cook the sweet potatoes, mixing them occasionally, until they are cooked and have a slight crunch to them.
5. Include salt and pepper as needed, depending on the situation.
6. During the time that the hash is being cooked, poach the eggs.
7. When serving, top the sweet potato hash with eggs that have been poached.
8. Decorate with fresh parsley as a garnish.

Per serving: Calories: 320kcal; Fat: 12g; Carbs: 45g; Protein: 10g; Sugar: 12g

LEGUMES RECIPES

16. Black Bean and Corn Salad

Preparation time: 10 minutes
Cooking time: 0 minutes
Servings: 4
Ingredients:

- 1 tin (15 oz) black beans, that is drained and washed
- 1 cup corn kernels
- 1 red bell pepper, cubed
- 1/2 red onion, finely cut into small bits
- 1/4 cup cilantro, cut into small bits
- Juice of 1 lime
- 2 tbsps olive oil
- 1 tsp cumin
- Salt and pepper as needed

Directions:

1. Blend cut into small bits red onion, black beans, corn, and cubed red bell pepper in a big bowl.
2. Blend the cumin, olive oil, and lime juice in a small bowl.
3. Cover the bean mixture with the dressing and toss to blend.
4. Flavor with pepper and salt as needed.
5. let your food cool in the fridge for nearly half an hour.

Per serving: Calories: 220kcal; Fat: 8g; Carbs: 32g; Protein: 8g; Sugar: 4g

17. Three Bean Salad with Lemon Dressing

Preparation time: 15 minutes
Cooking time: 0 minutes
Servings: 4
Ingredients:

- 1 tin (15 oz) kidney beans, that is drained and washed
- 1 tin (15 oz) black beans, that is drained and washed
- 1 tin (15 oz) garbanzo beans (chickpeas), that is drained and washed
- 1/2 red onion, finely cut into small bits
- 1/2 cup fresh parsley, cut into small bits
- Zest and juice of 2 lemons
- 3 tbsps olive oil
- Salt and pepper as needed

Directions:

1. Put the kidney beans, black beans, garbanzo beans, cut into small bits parsley, and red onion in a big bowl.
2. Blend the lemon zest, lemon juice, and olive oil in a small bowl.
3. Drizzle the beans with the dressing and shake to cover.
4. Flavor with pepper and salt as needed.
5. Prior to presenting, let your food cool in the fridge for nearly half an hour.

Per serving: Calories: 320kcal; Fat: 12g; Carbs: 40g; Protein: 15g; Sugar: 5g

18. White Bean and Kale Stew

Preparation time: 15 minutes
Cooking time: 25 minutes
Servings: 4
Ingredients:

- 2 cans (15 oz each) white beans, that is drained and washed

- 1 bunch kale, stems taken out & leaves cut into small bits
- 1 onion, finely cut into small bits
- 2 carrots, cubed
- 2 pieces garlic, crushed
- 4 cups vegetable broth (low sodium)
- 1 tsp dried thyme
- Salt and pepper as needed
- 1 tbsp olive oil

Directions:

1. Warm the olive oil in a big pot to a middling temp.
2. Include the cut into small bits onions and heat until they become tender.
3. Cook the cubed carrots and crushed garlic for a further 2 minutes.
4. Include the white beans, kale, and dried thyme in the vegetable broth.
5. Bring to a boil, lower the heat, and simmer the vegetables for 20 to 25 minutes, or until they are soft.
6. Flavor with pepper and salt as needed.
7. Present warm.

Per serving: Calories: 280kcal; Fat: 4g; Carbs: 50g; Protein: 15g; Sugar: 6g

19. Black-Eyed Pea and Vegetable Medley

Preparation time: 15 minutes
Cooking time: 25 minutes
Servings: 4
Ingredients:

- 2 cans (15 oz each) black-eyed peas, that is drained and washed
- 1 zucchini, cubed
- 1 red bell pepper, cubed

- 1 cup cherry tomatoes, divided
- 1/2 red onion, finely cut into small bits
- 2 pieces garlic, crushed
- 2 tbsps olive oil
- 1 tsp cumin
- 1/2 tsp smoked paprika
- Salt and pepper as needed
- Fresh cilantro for garnish

Directions:

1. Warm the olive oil in a big skillet to a middling temp.
2. Include the cut into small bits red onion and smashed garlic, and sauté until the onion becomes tender.
3. Cook the vegetables until they are crisp-tender by mixing in the cubed zucchini, red bell pepper, and cherry tomatoes.
4. Stir in the black-eyed peas, cumin, smoked paprika, salt, and pepper. Continue mixing until everything is thoroughly blended and heated.
5. Use fresh cilantro as a garnish.
6. Present warm.

Per serving: Calories: 280kcal; Fat: 8g; Carbs: 40g; Protein: 14g; Sugar: 6g

20. Pinto Bean and Vegetable Chili

Preparation time: 15 minutes
Cooking time: 30 minutes
Servings: 6
Ingredients:

- 2 cans (15 oz each) pinto beans, that is drained and washed
- 1 onion, finely cut into small bits
- 2 bell peppers, cubed

- 2 carrots, cubed
- 2 pieces garlic, crushed
- 1 tin (14 oz) cubed tomatoes
- 1 tin (6 oz) tomato paste
- 4 cups vegetable broth (low sodium)
- 2 tsps chili powder
- 1 tsp cumin
- Salt and pepper as needed
- 2 tbsps olive oil
- Optional toppings: shredded cheese, cut into small bits green onions, sour cream

Directions:

1. Bring the olive oil to a temp. just in the middle of your big pot.
2. Include cut into small bits onions, then continue to sauté until they have become more pliable.
3. Include the smashed garlic, cubed bell peppers, and cubed carrots, and continue to simmer for an extra two minutes while it is mixing.
4. The fourth step is to incorporate cubed tomatoes, tomato paste, pinto beans, vegetable broth, chili powder, cumin, salt, and pepper into the mixture.
5. Bring to a boil, then decrease the temp. to a simmer for twenty to thirty minutes.
6. Make any necessary adjustments to the flavoring.
7. Before serving, ensure that the dish is hot and garnish it with shredded cheese, cut into small bits green onions, and a dollop of sour cream, if necessary.

Per serving: Calories: 320kcal; Fat: 8g; Carbs: 50g; Protein: 15g; Sugar: 8g

21. Quinoa and Black Bean Bowl

Preparation time: 15 minutes
Cooking time: 15 minutes
Servings: 4
Ingredients:

- 1 cup quinoa, washed
- 2 cups water
- 1 tin (15 oz) black beans, that is drained and washed
- 1 cup corn kernels
- 1 avocado, cubed
- 1/4 cup red onion, finely cut into small bits
- 1/4 cup fresh cilantro, cut into small bits
- Juice of 1 lime
- Salt and pepper as needed

Directions:

1. Warm the water and quinoa together in the pot you have. To cook the quinoa, bring to a boil, then decrease the temp. to a simmer, cover, and continue cooking for 15 minutes.
2. In a big bowl, blend the quinoa that has been cooked previously, the black beans, the corn, the cubed avocado, the cut into small bits red onion, and the cut into small bits cilantro.
3. Include lime juice and stir to incorporate, then drizzle with lime juice.
4. Include salt and pepper as needed, depending on the situation.
5. Serve either warm or cold.

Per serving: Calories: 320kcal; Fat: 10g; Carbs: 50g; Protein: 12g; Sugar: 2g

22. Garbanzo Bean Salad with Cherry Tomatoes

Preparation time: 10 minutes
Cooking time: 0 minutes
Servings: 4
Ingredients:

- 2 cans (15 oz each) garbanzo beans, that is drained and washed
- 1 cup cherry tomatoes, divided
- 1/2 red onion, finely cut into small bits
- 1/4 cup fresh parsley, cut into small bits
- 2 tbsps olive oil
- 1 tbsp red wine vinegar
- 1 tsp Dijon mustard
- Salt and pepper as needed

Directions:

1. Begin by combining the garbanzo beans, cherry tomatoes that have been separated, cut into small bits red onion, and fresh parsley that has been cut into small bits in the big bowl.
2. In a small bowl, blend the following components: pepper, salt, olive oil, red wine vinegar, and Dijon mustard. Whisk until fully combined.
3. Put the dressing on top of the salad, and then toss it to evenly coat it.
4. Serve either cold or at room temp.

Per serving: Calories: 280kcal; Fat: 12g; Carbs: 30g; Protein: 15g; Sugar: 5g

23. Roasted Chickpea Snack

Preparation time: 10 minutes
Cooking time: 30 minutes
Servings: 4

Ingredients:

- 2 cans (15 oz each) chickpeas, that is drained and washed
- 2 tbsps olive oil
- 1 tsp ground cumin
- 1 tsp smoked paprika
- 1/2 tsp garlic powder
- Salt and pepper as needed

Directions:

1. While the oven is warming up at 400 deg.F, prepare your baking sheet by lining it with parchment paper.
2. Place chickpeas in a bowl and include salt, olive oil, cumin, smoked paprika, garlic powder, and pepper. Toss the chickpeas until they are evenly covered with the flavorings.
3. Organize the chickpeas in a single layer throughout the baking sheet that has been prepared.
4. Roast in an oven that has been preheated for 25 to 30 minutes while shaking the pan halfway through the cooking process.
5. Before presenting it, wait for it to cool down.

Per serving: Calories: 220kcal; Fat: 8g; Carbs: 30g; Protein: 10g; Sugar: 4g

24. Green Bean Almondine

Preparation time: 15 minutes
Cooking time: 10 minutes
Servings: 4
Ingredients:

- 1 lb green beans, trimmed
- 2 tbsps cut almonds
- 2 tbsps olive oil

- 2 pieces garlic, crushed
- 1 tbsp lemon juice
- Salt and pepper as needed
- Fresh parsley for garnish

Directions:

1. Steam or blanch the green beans for around 5 minutes, or until they are crisp-tender. After draining, put away the contents.
2. Toast the almonds into a golden brown color in your skillet at a temp. that is somewhere in the middle.
3. In a skillet, warm the olive oil, include the crushed garlic, and then sauté the mixture until it becomes aromatic.
4. Include the green beans that have been cooked to the skillet and let them stir in the oil that has been infused with garlic.
5. Include a drizzle of lemon juice and flavor with salt and pepper. Sprinkle with salt.
6. Transfer to a serving plate, flavor with toasted almonds, and finish with fresh parsley as a garnish.
7. Serve at a warm temp.

Per serving: Calories: 120kcal; Fat: 8g; Carbs: 10g; Protein: 3g; Sugar: 3g

- 1/2 red onion, finely cut into small bits
- 1/4 cup Kalamata olives, cut
- 1/4 cup feta cheese, crumbled
- 2 tbsps extra-virgin olive oil
- 1 tbsp red wine vinegar
- 1 tsp dried oregano
- Salt and pepper as needed
- Fresh parsley for garnish

Directions:

1. In a big bowl, include chicken lentils that have been cooked, sliced cucumber, cherry tomatoes that have been separated, cut into small bits red onion, Kalamata olives that have been cut, and crumbled feta cheese.
2. In a small bowl, blend the following components: pepper, dried oregano, olive oil, and red wine vinegar. Whisk together until combined.
3. Pour the dressing over the lentil mixture, and then toss it to be evenly coated.
4. Decorate with fresh parsley as a garnish.
5. May be served cold or at room temp.

Per serving: Calories: 280kcal; Fat: 12g; Carbs: 30g; Protein: 15g; Sugar: 5g

25. *Mediterranean Lentil Salad*

Preparation time: 15 minutes
Cooking time: 20 minutes (for lentils)
Servings: 4
Ingredients:

- 1 cup dry green or brown lentils, that is cooked
- 1 cucumber, cubed
- 1 cup cherry tomatoes, divided

PASTA AND CARBOHYDRATES RECIPES

26. Cauliflower Fried Rice with Shrimp

Preparation time: 15 minutes

Cooking time: 15 minutes

Servings: 4

Ingredients:

- 1 head cauliflower, grated or processed into rice-sized pieces
- 1 lb shrimp, skinned and deveined
- 2 cups mixed vegetables (peas, carrots, corn)
- 2 pieces garlic, crushed
- 2 tbsps soy sauce (low-sodium)
- 1 tbsp sesame oil
- 2 green onions, cut
- 2 eggs, beaten (optional)
- Sesame seeds for garnish

Directions:

1. Bring the amount of sesame oil to a med-high temp. in a big wok or skillet.
2. Include the shrimp, and then boil them until they are pink and opaque. First, remove the shrimp from the pan, and then put them away.
3. Garlic that has been crushed and a variety of veggies should be placed in the same pan for 3 to 5 minutes and stir-fried.
4. When you have the veggies pushed to one side of the pan, pour the eggs that have been beaten into the other side of the pan. Until the eggs are done, scramble them.
5. Include the shrimp that has been cooked on the stove, the cauliflower rice, and the soy sauce to the pan. Continue to stir-fry for an extra 5-7 minutes, until the entire ingredients are mixed together and heated through.
6. Garnish with green onions that have been cut into small bits and sesame seeds.
7. Serve while still hot.

Per serving: Calories: 250kcal; Fat: 8g; Carbs: 20g; Protein: 25g; Sugar: 6g

27. Zucchini Noodles with Pesto and Cherry Tomatoes

Preparation time: 15 minutes

Cooking time: 5 minutes

Servings: 2

Ingredients:

- 4 medium-sized zucchinis, spiralized into noodles
- 1 cup cherry tomatoes, divided
- 1/4 cup pesto sauce (store-bought or homemade)
- 2 tbsps pine nuts, toasted
- Salt and pepper as needed
- Fresh basil leaves for garnish

Directions:

1. In a big skillet, sauté the zucchini noodles at a temp. that is somewhere in the middle for 3 to 5 minutes, or until they are just soft.
2. After cherry tomatoes have been added to the pan, continue to simmer for an extra 2 minutes.

3. The third step is to thoroughly coat the zucchini noodles and cherry tomatoes with pesto sauce by tossing them together.

4. Include salt and pepper as needed, depending on the situation.

5. Sprinkle the zucchini noodles with pine nuts that have been toasted and fresh basil leaves prior to presenting.

6. Present instantly.

Per serving: Calories: 250kcal; Fat: 20g; Carbs: 15g; Protein: 6g; Sugar: 7g

28. Sweet Potato and Black Bean Quesadilla

Preparation time: 20 minutes
Cooking time: 15 minutes
Servings: 2
Ingredients:

- 2 big whole wheat tortillas
- 1 medium-sized sweet potato, skinned and grated
- 1 tin (15 oz) black beans, that is drained and washed
- 1 cup shredded cheese (cheddar or Mexican blend)
- 1 tsp cumin
- 1/2 tsp chili powder
- Salt and pepper as needed
- Olive oil for cooking
- Greek yogurt and salsa for presenting

Directions:

1. Blend grated sweet potato, black beans, cumin, chili powder, salt, and pepper in a bowl. Mix well. Serve instantly.

2. Bring a non-stick skillet to a temp. that is not too hot and include a tortilla to the pan.

3. Distribute 50 percent of the combination consisting of sweet potatoes and black beans across fifty percent of the tortilla.

4. The fourth step is to sprinkle the tortilla with shredded cheese and then fold it in half.

5. Cook until the cheese is melted and the tortilla is golden brown on both sides with a golden brown color.

6. Repeat with the second tortilla.

7. Cut each quesadilla into wedges, and serve them with Greek yogurt and salsa on the side.

Per serving: Calories: 450kcal; Fat: 18g; Carbs: 55g; Protein: 18g; Sugar: 4g

29. Barley and Mushroom Risotto

Preparation time: 10 minutes
Cooking time: 40 minutes
Servings: 4
Ingredients:

- 1 cup pearl barley
- 4 cups vegetable broth (low sodium)
- 1 onion, finely cut into small bits
- 2 pieces garlic, crushed
- 8 oz mushrooms, cut
- 1/2 cup dry white wine (optional)
- 2 tbsps olive oil
- 1/4 cup Parmesan cheese, grated
- Salt and pepper as needed
- Fresh parsley for garnish

Directions:

1. Bring the olive oil to a temp. just in the middle of your pot.
2. Include cut into small bits onions, then continue to sauté until they have become more pliable.
3. Include the cut into small bits mushrooms and crushed garlic, and continue to sauté the mixture until the mushrooms release their moisture.
4. Include the pearl barley, then continue cooking for an extra 2-3 minutes, until it has a mild toasty flavor.
5. If using white wine, pour it in, and continue cooking until the majority of the liquid has been absorbed.
6. Start including the vegetable broth, one cup at a time, mixing it constantly, and then wait for each addition to be absorbed before adding the next one.
7. Proceed with this process until the barley is soft and creamy, which should take approximately 40 minutes.
8. Incorporate grated Parmesan cheese into the mixture, then flavor it with salt and pepper.
9. Include some fresh parsley as a garnish.
10. Serve while still hot.

Per serving: Calories: 280kcal; Fat: 10g; Carbs: 40g; Protein: 8g; Sugar: 4g

30. Edamame and Walnut Salad

Preparation time: 15 minutes
Cooking time: 0 minutes
Servings: 4
Ingredients:

- 2 cups edamame beans (cooked and shelled)
- 1/2 cup walnuts, cut into small bits
- 1 cup cherry tomatoes, divided
- 1/4 cup red onion, finely cut into small bits
- 2 tbsps olive oil
- 1 tbsp balsamic vinegar
- Salt and pepper as needed
- Fresh mint for garnis

Directions:

1. Put the split cherry tomatoes, edamame beans, finely cut red onion, and cut into small bits walnuts in the bowl.
2. Blend the balsamic vinegar and olive oil in a small basin.
3. Drizzle the salad with the dressing and toss to mix.
4. Flavor with pepper and salt as needed.
5. Prior to presenting, garnish with fresh mint.

Per serving: Calories: 280kcal; Fat: 18g; Carbs: 18g; Protein: 14g; Sugar: 4g

31. Hummus and Veggie Wrap

Preparation time: 10 minutes
Cooking time: 0 minutes
Servings: 2
Ingredients:

- 4 whole grain or whole wheat wraps
- 1 cup hummus (store-bought or homemade)
- 1 cup mixed veggies (e.g., bell peppers, cucumber, carrots), finely cut
- 1 cup fresh spinach or lettuce leaves
- Salt and pepper as needed

Directions:

1. Put the wraps in a flat position on the surface.
2. Spread equal parts of a quarter cup of hummus on each wrap.
3. Split the sliced vegetables and spinach or lettuce in a uniform manner on every wrap before presenting.
4. Include salt and pepper as needed, depending on the situation.
5. Fold the wraps in half lengthwise and then fold them again before cutting them in half.
6. Present instantly.

Per serving: Calories: 320kcal; Fat: 12g; Carbs: 45g; Protein: 10g; Sugar: 5g

32. *Chickpea and Spinach Curry*

Preparation time: 15 minutes
Cooking time: 20 minutes
Servings: 4
Ingredients:

- 1 tin (15 oz) chickpeas, that is drained and washed
- 1 onion, finely cut into small bits
- 2 tomatoes, cubed
- 3 cups fresh spinach
- 1 tin (14 oz) coconut milk (unsweetened)
- 2 tbsps curry powder
- 1 tsp cumin
- 1 tsp turmeric
- 1 tbsp olive oil
- Salt and pepper as needed

Directions:

1. Bring the olive oil to a temp. right in the middle of your big pan.
2. After adding cut into small bits onions, sauté them until they become more pliable.
3. After it has been cooking for an extra 2 minutes, stir in the curry powder, cumin, and turmeric.
4. Include cubed tomatoes, then continue to simmer until the tomatoes begin to get softer.
5. After pouring in the coconut milk, bring the mixture to a simmer.
6. Include chickpeas and fresh spinach, and simmer the mixture until the spinach has wilted before serving.
7. Include salt and pepper as needed, depending on the situation.
8. To present, put the curry on top of quinoa or brown rice.

Per serving: Calories: 350kcal; Fat: 20g; Carbs: 35g; Protein: 12g; Sugar: 5g

33. *Split Pea Soup with Carrots and Celery*

Preparation time: 15 minutes
Cooking time: 1 hour
Servings: 6
Ingredients:

- 2 cups split peas, washed
- 1 onion, cut into small bits
- 2 carrots, cubed
- 2 celery stalks, cubed
- 2 pieces garlic, crushed
- 8 cups vegetable broth (low sodium)
- 1 tsp dried thyme
- Salt and pepper as needed
- 1 tbsp olive oil

Directions:

1. Bring the olive oil to a temp. just in the middle of your big pot.
2. Include cut into small bits onions, then continue to sauté until they have become more pliable.
3. The third step is to include cubed carrots, cubed celery, and smashed garlic, and continue to sauté for an extra 2 minutes.
4. Pour in the vegetable broth, then include the dried thyme and split peas to the mixture.
5. Bring to a boil, then decrease the temp. but continue to simmer for one hour, or until the split peas are cooked.
6. Include salt and pepper as needed, depending on the situation.
7. Serve while still hot.

Per serving: Calories: 280kcal; Fat: 4g; Carbs: 45g; Protein: 15g; Sugar: 8g

34. *Lentil and Vegetable Stir-Fry*

Preparation time: 15 minutes
Cooking time: 20 minutes
Servings: 4
Ingredients:

- 1 cup dry lentils, washed then cooked
- 2 cups mixed vegetables (e.g., broccoli, bell peppers, snap peas), cut into small bits
- 1 onion, finely cut
- 2 pieces garlic, crushed
- 1/4 cup low-sodium soy sauce
- 1 tbsp sesame oil
- 1 tsp ginger, grated

- 2 green onions, cut
- Sesame seeds for garnish

Directions:

1. Bring the sesame oil temp. up to a medium-high level in your wok or big skillet.
2. Stir-frying for 1 to 2 minutes while adding cut into small bits onions and garlic that has been smashed.
3. Include a variety of veggies, start with lentils that have been cooked, and stir-fry the vegetables until they are tender but still crunchy.
4. Include grated ginger and pour in the soy sauce, then toss everything together until it is evenly distributed.
5. Cook for an extra 2 to 3 minutes.
6. Before delivering the dish, garnish it with green onions that have been sliced and sesame seeds.

Per serving: Calories: 320kcal; Fat: 8g; Carbs: 50g; Protein: 18g; Sugar: 4g

35. *Spinach and Ricotta Stuffed Bell Peppers*

Preparation time: 20 minutes
Cooking time: 30 minutes
Servings: 4
Ingredients:

- 4 bell peppers, divided and seeds taken out
- 1 cup quinoa, cooked
- 1 cup ricotta cheese
- 1 cup cut into small bits spinach
- 1/2 cup grated Parmesan cheese
- 2 pieces garlic, crushed

- 1 tsp dried Italian herbs (basil, oregano, thyme)
- Salt and pepper as needed
- 1 tin (14 oz) cubed tomatoes, drained
- 1/2 cup shredded mozzarella cheese
- Fresh basil for garnish

Directions:

1. Warm up your oven to 375 deg.F.
2. In a bowl, blend the quinoa that has been cooked, the ricotta cheese, the cut into small bits spinach, the grated Parmesan cheese, the smashed garlic, and the dried Italian herbs, which are flavored with salt and pepper.
3. Stuff the bell peppers that have been separated with the combination of quinoa and ricotta cheese.
4. Put the peppers that have been packed into the baking dish.
5. Place a layer of cut into small bits tomatoes and shredded mozzarella cheese on top of each pepper that has been packed.
6. Put the dish in an oven that has been preheated and bake for 25 to 30 minutes, or until the peppers are soft and the cheese is melted and bubbling.
7. Before delivering the dish, garnish it with plenty of fresh basil.

Per serving: Calories: 320kcal; Fat: 14g; Carbs: 35g; Protein: 15g; Sugar: 6g

36. *Bulgur Pilaf with Mixed Vegetables*

Preparation time: 15 minutes
Cooking time: 20 minutes
Servings: 4
Ingredients:

- 1 cup coarse bulgur
- 2 cups vegetable broth (low sodium)
- 1 onion, finely cut into small bits
- 1 carrot, cubed
- 1 zucchini, cubed
- 1 red bell pepper, cubed
- 2 tbsps olive oil
- 1 tsp ground cumin
- Salt and pepper as needed
- Fresh parsley for garnish

Directions:

1. Bring the olive oil to a temp. just in the middle of your pot.
2. Include cut into small bits onions, then continue to sauté until they have become more pliable.
3. Continue to sauté the mixture for an extra 5 minutes while mixing in cubed carrots, cubed zucchini, and cubed red bell pepper.
4. Include the bulgur to the pot and stir it occasionally so that it may coat the veggies.
5. Include ground cumin, salt, and pepper to the mixture, and then pour in the vegetable broth. Take a boil.
6. Decrease the temp., cover the pot, and begin to simmer the bulgur for fifteen to twenty minutes, or until it has become tender and has absorbed the liquid.
7. To finish, sprinkle the bulgur with some fresh parsley after you have fluffed it with a fork.
8. Serve at a warm.

Per serving: Calories: 280kcal; Fat: 10g; Carbs: 40g; Protein: 8g; Sugar: 5g

37. Whole Grain Penne with Roasted Vegetables

Preparation time: 15 minutes
Cooking time: 25 minutes
Servings: 4
Ingredients:

- 8 oz whole grain penne pasta
- 2 bell peppers, cut
- 1 zucchini, cut
- 1 eggplant, cubed
- 1 red onion, cut
- 3 tbsps olive oil
- 2 pieces garlic, crushed
- 1 tsp dried oregano
- Salt and pepper as needed
- Grated Parmesan cheese for garnish (optional)
- Fresh basil for garnish

Directions:

1. Warm up your oven to 400 deg.F.
2. Using a big baking sheet, blend the bell peppers, zucchini, eggplant, and red onion that have been cut into small bits into pieces with the following components: salt, olive oil, crushed garlic, dry oregano, and pepper.
3. Roast the veggies in an oven that has been preheated for 20 to 25 minutes, or until they are soft and have a light brown color.
4. In the meantime, while the veggies are roasting, prepare the whole grain penne pasta by the instructions on the package. Run off.
5. Blend the cooked spaghetti with the vegetables that have been roasted.
6. If you are using it, garnish with grated Parmesan cheese and fresh basil.

7. Serve at a warm temp.

Per serving: Calories: 350kcal; Fat: 12g; Carbs: 50g; Protein: 10g; Sugar: 5g

38. Butternut Squash and Sage Risotto

Preparation time: 15 minutes
Cooking time: 30 minutes
Servings: 4
Ingredients:

- 1 cup Arborio rice
- 1/2 butternut squash, skinned and cubed
- 1 onion, finely cut into small bits
- 2 pieces garlic, crushed
- 4 cups vegetable broth (low sodium)
- 1/2 cup dry white wine (optional)
- 2 tbsps olive oil
- 1 tbsp fresh sage, cut into small bits
- 1/4 cup Parmesan cheese, grated
- Salt and pepper as needed

Directions:

1. Bring the olive oil to a temp. just in the middle of your pot.
2. Include cut into small bits onions, then continue to sauté until they have become more pliable.
3. Sauté the Arborio rice and smashed garlic for two to three minutes while mixing the mixture.
4. After adding the butternut squash that has been cubed, continue to simmer the dish for an extra 5 minutes.
5. If using white wine, pour it in, and continue cooking until the majority of the liquid has been absorbed.

6. Start adding the vegetable broth, one cup at a time, mixing it constantly, and then wait for each addition to be absorbed before adding the next one.

7. For approximately 20 to 25 minutes, continue this process until the rice is creamy and then cooked until it is al dente.

8. Eighth, incorporate grated Parmesan cheese and fresh sage that has been cubed. Salt and pepper should be used to flavor.

9. Warm the food.

Per serving: Calories: 320kcal; Fat: 8g; Carbs: 55g; Protein: 6g; Sugar: 4g

39. *Spaghetti Squash with Marinara Sauce*

Preparation time: 10 minutes
Cooking time: 40 minutes
Servings: 4
Ingredients:

- 1 medium-sized spaghetti squash, divided and seeds taken out
- 2 cups marinara sauce (store-bought or homemade)
- 1 tbsp olive oil
- 1/4 cup fresh basil, cut into small bits
- Salt and pepper as needed
- Grated Parmesan cheese for garnish (optional)

Directions:

1. Warm up your oven to 375 deg.F.

2. Flavor the spaghetti squash with salt and pepper, then drizzle olive oil over the cut sides of the squash and flavor all over with salt.

3. Organize the squash halves on the baking sheet with the sliced side facing down.

4. Put the squash in the oven and bake for thirty to 40 minutes, or until it is tender and can be easily shredded with a fork.

5. With the help of a fork, scrape the flesh of the squash into strands that resemble spaghetti.

6. To prepare the spaghetti squash, warm the marinara sauce in a skillet and then pour it over the squash.

7. Toss the squash in the sauce so that it is well coated, and then garnish it with fresh basil that has been cut into small bits and, if necessary, grated Parmesan cheese.

8. Serve warm.

Per serving: Calories: 150kcal; Fat: 6g; Carbs: 20g; Protein: 3g; Sugar: 8g

40. *Cabbage and Beef Stir-Fry with Brown Rice*

Preparation time: 15 minutes
Cooking time: 15 minutes
Servings: 4
Ingredients:

- 1 lb lean ground beef
- 4 cups green cabbage, shredded
- 1 carrot, julienned
- 1 bell pepper, cut
- 2 tbsps soy sauce (low-sodium)
- 1 tbsp oyster sauce
- 1 tbsp sesame oil
- 2 pieces garlic, crushed
- 1 tbsp ginger, grated

- 4 cups cooked brown rice
-

Directions:

1. Brown the ground beef in a big wok or skillet utilizing a med-high temp.
2. After sautéing for a couple of minutes, include the grated ginger and crushed garlic to the mixture.
3. Put the shredded cabbage, carrots that have been julienned, and bell peppers that have been cut into small bits into the wok. For 5-7 minutes, stir-fry the vegetables until they are soft but still crunchy.
4. Blend the soy sauce, oyster sauce, and sesame oil in the medium-sized bowl you have available to you.
5. Pour the sauce over the beef and vegetable mixture, and then toss it to ensure that it is evenly coated.
6. Put the stir-fry on top of the brown rice that has been prepared.

Per serving: Calories: 380kcal; Fat: 15g; Carbs: 40g; Protein: 20g; Sugar: 5g

41. Brown Rice Stir-Fry with Tofu and Vegetables

Preparation time: 15 minutes
Cooking time: 20 minutes
Servings: 4
Ingredients:

- 2 cups cooked brown rice
- 1 block firm tofu, pressed and cubed
- 2 cups mixed vegetables (broccoli, bell peppers, snap peas)
- 3 tbsps low-sodium soy sauce
- 1 tbsp sesame oil

- 2 pieces garlic, crushed
- 1 tsp ginger, grated
- 2 green onions, cut
- Sesame seeds for garnish

Directions:

1. Bring the amount of sesame oil to a med-high temp. in a big wok or skillet.
2. Include cubed tofu, and stir-fry it until it is golden brown on all sides from the bottom up.
3. After sautéing for a couple of minutes, include the grated ginger and crushed garlic to the mixture.
4. Include a variety of veggies to the wok, followed by brown rice that has been partially cooked, and stir everything together.
5. Pour in the soy sauce and continue to stir-fry the vegetables until they are cooked but still have a crisp texture.
6. Garnish with green onions that have been cut into small bits and sesame seeds.
7. Serve while still hot.

Per serving: Calories: 320kcal; Fat: 12g; Carbs: 40g; Protein: 15g; Sugar: 3g

42. Whole Wheat Pasta with Tomato & Basil Sauce

Preparation time: 15 minutes
Cooking time: 15 minutes
Servings: 4
Ingredients:

- 8 oz whole wheat pasta
- 2 cups cherry tomatoes, divided
- 3 pieces garlic, crushed
- 2 tbsps olive oil

- 1/4 tsp red pepper flakes
- Salt and pepper as needed
- Fresh basil leaves for garnish
- Grated Parmesan cheese (optional)

Directions:

1. Prepare the whole wheat pasta in accordance with the instructions provided on the package. After draining, put away the contents.
2. Bring the olive oil to a temp. that is on the middle in your skillet.
3. After adding the smashed garlic, sauté it for a couple of minutes until it becomes aromatic.
4. Cherry tomatoes, red pepper flakes (if using), salt, and pepper should be included in the fourth step. Cook the tomatoes for 5-7 minutes, or until they become tender and release their juices.
5. Toss the pasta that has been cooked throughout the tomato and basil sauce.
6. To finish, garnish with fresh basil leaves and, if desired, sprinkle with grated Parmesan cheese.
7. Serve at a warm temp.

Per serving: Calories: 300kcal; Fat: 8g; Carbs: 50g; Protein: 10g; Sugar: 4g

43. Eggplant Lasagna with Ground Turkey

Preparation time: 20 minutes
Cooking time: 45 minutes
Servings: 6
Ingredients:

- 1 big eggplant, cut lengthwise
- 1 lb ground turkey
- 1 onion, finely cut into small bits
- 2 pieces garlic, crushed
- 1 tin (14 oz) crushed tomatoes
- 1 tin (6 oz) tomato paste
- 1 tsp dried basil
- 1 tsp dried oregano
- Salt and pepper as needed
- 2 cups part-skim ricotta cheese
- 1 cup shredded mozzarella cheese
- 1/2 cup grated Parmesan cheese
- Fresh basil for garnish

Directions:

1. Warm up your oven to 375 deg.F.
2. To brown the ground turkey, heat it in your skillet at a temp. that is somewhere in the middle. Put in some cut into small bits onions and crushed garlic, and sauté them until they become more pliable.
3. Include crushed tomatoes, tomato paste, dried basil, dried oregano, salt, and pepper to the mixture and stir to blend. Simmer for 10 to 15 minutes.
4. Ricotta cheese, mozzarella cheese, and Parmesan cheese should be mixed together in a separate bowl.
5. Arrange cubed eggplant, turkey-tomato sauce, and ricotta cheese mixture in alternating layers in a baking dish that has been buttered. Maintain this process until the entire components have been utilized, culminating with a layer of cheese on top.
6. Put the lasagna in an oven that has been preheated and bake it for 30 minutes or until it is bubbling and brown.
7. Before delivering the dish, garnish it with plenty of fresh basil.

Per serving: Calories: 350kcal; Fat: 15g; Carbs: 25g; Protein: 25g; Sugar: 8g

44. Whole Wheat Couscous Salad with Chickpeas

Preparation time: 15 minutes

Cooking time: 10 minutes

Servings: 4

Ingredients:

- 1 cup whole wheat couscous
- 1 tin (15 oz) chickpeas, drained and washed
- 1 cucumber, cubed
- 1 cup cherry tomatoes, divided
- 1/4 cup red onion, finely cut into small bits
- 1/4 cup fresh parsley, cut into small bits
- 2 tbsps olive oil
- 1 tbsp lemon juice
- 1 tsp ground cumin
- Salt and pepper as needed

Directions:

1. Cook the whole wheat couscous as per to the guidelines on the package.
2. In a big bowl, blend the cooked couscous, the chickpeas, the cubed cucumber, the cherry tomatoes, the cut red onion, and the small bits of fresh parsley.
3. Transfer the ground cumin, lemon juice, olive oil, and salt and pepper to a small bowl and whisk the entire components together.
4. Put the dressing on top of the couscous mixture, and then toss to evenly distribute the dressing.

5. May be served cold or at room temp.

Per serving: Calories: 320kcal; Fat: 10g; Carbs: 50g; Protein: 10g; Sugar: 5g

45. Broccoli and Cheddar Stuffed Baked Potatoes

Preparation time: 15 minutes

Cooking time: 1 hour

Servings: 4

Ingredients:

- 4 big baking potatoes
- 2 cups broccoli florets, steamed
- 1 cup shredded cheddar cheese
- 1/2 cup Greek yogurt (plain)
- 2 tbsps cut into small bits chives
- Salt and pepper as needed

Directions:

1. Warm up your oven to 400 deg.F.
2. Using a fork, pierce each potato, and then bake them for 45 to 60 minutes, or until they are soft.
3. Prepare each roasted potato by making a slit in the top and using a fork to fluff the insides of the potato.
4. Blend steamed broccoli, shredded cheddar cheese, Greek yogurt, cut into small bits chives, salt, and pepper in a bowl. Continue mixing until everything is evenly distributed.
5. Place a single layer of the broccoli and cheddar mixture inside of each baked potato.
6. Return the stuffed potatoes to the oven and bake them until the cheese has melted and become bubbling.
7. Serve while still hot.

Per serving: Calories: 300kcal; Fat: 8g; Carbs: 50g; Protein: 10g; Sugar: 3g

SAUCES RECIPES

46. Roasted Red Pepper Sauce

Preparation time: 15 minutes

Cooking time: 20 minutes

Servings: 8 (2 tbsps per serving)

Ingredients:

- 2 red bell peppers, roasted and skinned
- 1 tbsp olive oil
- 2 pieces garlic, crushed
- 1/4 tsp crushed red pepper flakes
- Salt and pepper as needed
- 1 tbsp balsamic vinegar
- 1/4 cup fresh basil, cut into small bits

Directions:

1. If you want the skin of the red bell peppers to be charred, roast them over an open flame or broil them in the oven.
2. Put the roasted peppers in the bowl, cover them with plastic wrap, and allow them to steam for 10 minutes. To prepare the flesh, first get rid of the seeds and then take off the skin.
3. Raise the temp. of the olive oil in the skillet to a medium level. When you include the crushed garlic, sauté it for one to two minutes until it becomes aromatic.
4. Include the cut into small bits roasted red peppers, crushed red pepper flakes (if you would want to use them), salt, and pepper to the mixture. 5-7 minutes of cooking time.
5. Put the mixture in a blender and include the balsamic vinegar and fresh basil to achieve the desired consistency. Blend until it is completely smooth.
6. Adjust the flavoring if it is required, and then put the container in the fridge, making sure it is sealed.

Per serving: Calories: 30kcal; Fat: 2g; Carbs: 3g; Protein: 1g; Sugar: 2g

47. Cilantro Lime Vinaigrette

Preparation time: 10 minutes

Cooking time: 0 minutes

Servings: 8 (2 tbsps per serving)

Ingredients:

- 1/2 cup fresh cilantro, cut into small bits
- 1/4 cup olive oil
- 2 tbsps lime juice
- 1 tsp honey or a sugar substitute
- 1 piece garlic, crushed
- Salt and pepper as needed

Directions:

1. Put the cut into small bits cilantro, olive oil, lime juice, honey (or a sugar replacement), crushed garlic, salt, and pepper into a mixer and mix until everything is distributed evenly.
2. Blend until it is completely smooth and completely blended.
3. Make any necessary adjustments to the sweetness and flavoring.
4. Put in the fridge in the container that you have sealed.
5. Give it a good shake before being presented.

Per serving: Calories: 80kcal; Fat: 7g; Carbs: 4g; Protein: 0g; Sugar: 2g

48. Garlic and Herb Marinara Sauce

Preparation time: 15 minutes
Cooking time: 30 minutes
Servings: 8 (1/2 cup per serving)
Ingredients:

- 2 tbsps olive oil
- 1 onion, finely cut into small bits
- 3 pieces garlic, crushed
- 1 tin (28 oz) crushed tomatoes
- 1 tin (14 oz) cubed tomatoes
- 2 tsps dried oregano
- 1 tsp dried basil
- 1/2 tsp dried thyme
- Salt and pepper as needed
- 1 tsp sugar or sugar substitute (optional)

Directions:

1. Bring the olive oil to a temp. just in the middle in your saucepan. The onions should be cubed and then sautéed until they become softer.
2. After adding the garlic that has been crushed, keep sauteing for a couple of minutes.
3. Step three: Include cubed tomatoes and crushed tomatoes to the mixture. In order to mix, stir.
4. Incorporate dried oregano, dried basil, dried thyme, as well as salt and pepper into the mixture. Give it a good stir.
5. Bring the sauce to a simmer, and then allow it to boil for twenty to thirty minutes while mixing it occasionally.
6. A sample of the flavoring should be taken, and any necessary modifications should be made. In order to achieve a balance of acidity, sugar or a sugar substitute should be included.
7. Take the sauce off the heat once it has reached the desired consistency.
8. Use it right away, or wait until it has cooled down before putting it in the fridge in the container that you covered.

Per serving: Calories: 70kcal; Fat: 3g; Carbs: 10g; Protein: 2g; Sugar: 6g

49. Avocado Lime Sauce

Preparation time: 10 minutes
Cooking time: 0 minutes
Servings: 8 (2 tbsps per serving)
Ingredients:

- 2 ripe avocados, skinned and pitted
- 1/4 cup fresh cilantro, cut into small bits
- 1 piece garlic, crushed
- Juice of 2 limes
- 1/4 cup Greek yogurt (plain, non-fat)
- Salt and pepper as needed

Directions:

1. Put ripe avocados, cut into small bits cilantro, crushed garlic, lime juice, Greek yogurt, salt, and pepper into a mixer and mix until everything is evenly distributed.
2. Whip until it is silky smooth and creamy.
3. Adjust the flavoring as needed as necessary.
4. Put in the fridge in the container that you have sealed.
5. Use this sauce as a dip or as a sauce for chicken or fish that has been grilled.

Per serving: Calories: 60kcal; Fat: 5g; Carbs: 4g; Protein: 2g; Sugar: 0g

50. Greek Yogurt and Dill Dressing

Preparation time: 10 minutes
Cooking time: 0 minutes
Servings: 8 (2 tbsps per serving)
Ingredients:

- 1 cup Greek yogurt (plain, non-fat)
- 2 tbsps fresh dill, cut into small bits
- 1 tbsp lemon juice
- 1 piece garlic, crushed
- Salt and pepper as needed

Directions:

1. Put the Greek yogurt, salt, fresh dill that has been cut into small bits, lemon juice, smashed garlic, and pepper into a bowl and mix them together.
2. Stir the mixture until it is completely blended.
3. Adjust the flavoring as needed as necessary.
4. Put it in the fridge until you are ready to use it.
5. Give it a thorough stir prior to presenting.

Per serving: Calories: 25kcal; Fat: 0g; Carbs: 3g; Protein: 3g; Sugar: 2g

51. Mango Salsa with Cucumber

Preparation time: 15 minutes
Cooking time: 0 minutes
Servings: 8 (1/4 cup per serving)
Ingredients:

- 1 big mango, skinned, pitted, and cubed
- 1/2 English cucumber, cubed
- 1/4 cup red onion, finely cut into small bits
- 1/4 cup cilantro, cut into small bits
- 1 jalapeño, seeds taken out and crushed (optional)
- Juice of 2 limes
- Salt and pepper as needed

Directions:

1. In a bowl, include the following components: cubed mango, cubed cucumber, cut into small bits red onion, cut into small bits cilantro, crushed jalapeño (if using), lime juice, salt, and pepper.
2. Mix carefully until everything is completely blended.
3. Put it in the fridge for close to half an hour before showing it to the audience.
4. Use it as a reviving topping for your grilled chicken or fish, or use it as a dip.

Per serving: Calories: 25kcal; Fat: 0g; Carbs: 6g; Protein: 0g; Sugar: 4g

52. Avocado Cilantro Lime Crema

Preparation time: 10 minutes
Cooking time: 0 minutes
Servings: 8 (2 tbsps per serving)
Ingredients:

- 1 ripe avocado, skinned and pitted
- 1/4 cup Greek yogurt (plain, non-fat)
- 1 tbsp fresh cilantro, cut into small bits
- Juice of 1 lime
- 1 piece garlic, crushed
- Salt and pepper as needed

Directions:

1. Put the ripe avocado, Greek yogurt, cut into small bits fresh cilantro, lime juice, crushed garlic, salt, and pepper into a mixer and beat until everything is combined.

2. Whip until it is silky smooth and creamy.

3. Adjust the flavoring as needed as necessary.

4. Store the contents of your container in the fridge until you are ready to utilize them.

5. In addition to serving as a dip, you can use it as a creamy topping for tacos or grilled chicken.

Per serving: Calories: 50kcal; Fat: 4g; Carbs: 3g; Protein: 1g; Sugar: 1g

53. Apple Cider Vinegar Coleslaw Dressing

Preparation time: 10 minutes
Cooking time: 0 minutes
Servings: 6 (2 tbsps per serving)
Ingredients:

- 1/4 cup apple cider vinegar
- 2 tbsps Dijon mustard
- 1 tbsp honey or a sugar substitute
- 2 tbsps olive oil
- Salt and pepper as needed
- 4 cups shredded cabbage and carrots (pre-packaged coleslaw mix)

Directions:

1. In a small bowl, blend the apple cider vinegar, Dijon mustard, honey (or a sugar replacement), olive oil, salt, and pepper by first whisking the entire components together.

2. In a big bowl, put the shredded cabbage and carrots that you have prepared.

3. Put the dressing on top of the cabbage mixture, and then toss it until it is evenly coated.

4. In order to allow the flavors to blend, put the dish in the fridge for a total of 30 minutes before presenting it.

5. Serve as a side dish while it is cooled.

Per serving: Calories: 60kcal; Fat: 4g; Carbs: 6g; Protein: 1g; Sugar: 4g

54. Honey Mustard Glazed Carrots

Preparation time: 10 minutes
Cooking time: 15 minutes
Servings: 4
Ingredients:

- 1 lb baby carrots
- 2 tbsps Dijon mustard
- 1 tbsp honey or a sugar substitute
- 1 tbsp olive oil
- Salt and pepper as needed
- Fresh parsley for garnish (optional)

Directions:

1. Baby carrots should be steamed or boiled until they are just soft.

2. In a small bowl, blend the Dijon mustard, honey (or sugar replacement), olive oil, salt, and pepper by whisking them together.

3. To ensure that the carrots are evenly coated, toss them with the honey mustard glaze after they have been cooked.

4. If necessary, decoratively garnish with fresh parsley.

5. Serve while still warm.

Per serving: Calories: 90kcal; Fat: 4g; Carbs: 14g; Protein: 1g; Sugar: 9g

55. Greek Tzatziki Sauce

Preparation time: 10 minutes
Cooking time: 0 minutes
Servings: 8 (2 tbsps per serving)
Ingredients:

- 1 cup Greek yogurt (plain, non-fat)
- 1 cucumber, grated and drained
- 2 pieces garlic, crushed
- 1 tbsp fresh dill, cut into small bits
- 1 tbsp olive oil
- 1 tsp lemon juice
- Salt and pepper as needed

Directions:

1. In a bowl, include the following components: Greek yogurt, grated and drained cucumber, crushed garlic, fresh dill that has been cut into small bits, olive oil, lemon juice, salt, and pepper.
2. Mix till everything is completely blended.
3. Adjust the flavoring as needed as necessary.
4. Store the contents of your container in the fridge until you are ready to utilize them.
5. Serve as a sauce for grilled chicken, or as a sauce for gyros.

Per serving: Calories: 40kcal; Fat: 3g; Carbs: 2g; Protein: 2g; Sugar: 1g

56. Lemon Dijon Mustard Dressing

Preparation time: 5 minutes
Cooking time: 0 minutes
Servings: 8 (2 tbsps per serving)
Ingredients:

- 3 tbsps olive oil
- 2 tbsps Dijon mustard
- 1 tbsp lemon juice
- 1 tsp honey or a sugar substitute
- 1 piece garlic, crushed
- Salt and pepper as needed

Directions:

1. In a small bowl, blend the following components: olive oil, Dijon mustard, lemon juice, honey (or a sugar replacement), crushed garlic, salt, and pepper. Whisk until they are combined.
2. Make any necessary adjustments to the sweetness and flavoring.
3. Put in the fridge in the container that you have sealed.
4. Give it a good shake before you present it.

Per serving: Calories: 60kcal; Fat: 6g; Carbs: 2g; Protein: 0g; Sugar: 1g

57. Balsamic Glazed Brussels Sprouts

Preparation time: 10 minutes
Cooking time: 20 minutes
Servings: 4
Ingredients:

- 1 lb Brussels sprouts, trimmed and divided

- 2 tbsps olive oil
- 2 tbsps balsamic vinegar
- 1 tbsp honey or a sugar substitute
- Salt and pepper as needed
- 2 tbsps cut into small bits fresh parsley

Directions:

1. Warm up your oven to 400 deg.F.
2. Put the Brussels sprouts in a bowl and include the olive oil, balsamic vinegar, honey (or equivalent sugar alternative), salt, and pepper. Toss to blend.
3. Organize the Brussels sprouts in a single layer on the baking sheet you have prepared.
4. Rotate the items in an oven that has been preheated for 15 to 20 minutes, or until they have a golden brown color and a crisp outside.
5. After taking out the dish from the oven, if necessary, sprinkle it with fresh parsley that has been cut into small bits.
6. Serve quickly.

Per serving: Calories: 90kcal; Fat: 5g; Carbs: 11g; Protein: 3g; Sugar: 5g

58. Tahini Yogurt Sauce

Preparation time: 10 minutes
Cooking time: 0 minutes
Servings: 8 (2 tbsps per serving)
Ingredients:

- 1/2 cup Greek yogurt (plain, non-fat)
- 2 tbsps tahini
- 1 tbsp lemon juice
- 1 piece garlic, crushed
- Salt and pepper as needed
- Water (optional, to thin the sauce)

Directions:

1. The first step is to blend Greek yogurt, tahini, lemon juice, smashed garlic, salt, and pepper in a bowl and whisk them together well.
2. If you find that the sauce is too dense, a small amount of water should be added and whisked until the correct consistency is achieved.
3. Adjust the flavoring as needed as necessary.
4. Store the contents of your container in the fridge until you are ready to utilize them.
5. Give it a thorough stir prior to presenting.

Per serving: Calories: 50kcal; Fat: 4g; Carbs: 2g; Protein: 2g; Sugar: 0g

59. Sesame Ginger Soy Sauce

Preparation time: 10 minutes
Cooking time: 0 minutes
Servings: 8 (2 tbsps per serving)
Ingredients:

- 1/4 cup low-sodium soy sauce
- 1 tbsp sesame oil
- 1 tbsp rice vinegar
- 1 tbsp fresh ginger, grated
- 1 tbsp green onions, finely cut into small bits
- 1 tsp sesame seeds (optional)

Directions:

1. In a bowl, blend low-sodium soy sauce, sesame oil, rice vinegar, grated fresh ginger, and cut into small bits green onions by whisking the entire components together.

2. If you are using sesame seeds, stir them in.

3. Adjust the flavoring as needed as necessary.

4. Put it in the fridge in the container that you have sealed.

5. You may use it as a marinade for your grilled meats, as a dipping sauce for sushi, or as a spring roll sauce.

Per serving: Calories: 25kcal; Fat: 2g; Carbs: 1g; Protein: 1g; Sugar: 0g

as a topping for yogurt, provide this sauce.

Per serving: Calories: 40kcal; Fat: 0g; Carbs: 10g; Protein: 0g; Sugar: 7g

60. Cranberry Orange Relish

Preparation time: 10 minutes

Cooking time: 0 minutes

Servings: 8 (2 tbsps per serving)

Ingredients:

- 1 cup fresh cranberries
- 1 orange, skinned and segmented
- 1/4 cup honey or a sugar substitute
- 1 tbsp orange zest
- 1/4 cup fresh mint leaves (optional)

Directions:

1. Put the fresh cranberries, an orange that has been skinned and segmented, honey (or a sugar alternative), and orange zest into a blender (or other similar device).

2. Continue to pulse the mixture until it achieves the consistency that you want.

3. If you are using fresh mint leaves, stir them in.

4. Before showing it to the audience, put it in the fridge for roughly half an hour.

5. For a tangy and refreshing condiment that may be used on roasted meats or

VEGGIES RECIPES

61. Roasted Garlic Parmesan Brussels Sprouts

Preparation time: 10 minutes
Cooking time: 25 minutes
Servings: 4
Ingredients:

- 1 lb Brussels sprouts, trimmed and divided
- 2 tbsps olive oil
- 3 pieces garlic, crushed
- 2 tbsps Parmesan cheese, grated
- Salt and pepper as needed
- 1 tbsp fresh parsley, cut into small bits

Directions:

1. Warm up your oven to 400 deg.F.
2. The Brussels sprouts should be tossed in a basin with the following components: salt, olive oil, crushed garlic, Parmesan cheese, and pepper.
3. Organize the Brussels sprouts in a single layer on the baking sheet you have prepared.
4. Roast in an oven that has been preheated for 20 to 25 minutes, or until they have a golden brown color and their edges have become crispy.
5. Take out the dish from the oven and, if necessary, sprinkle it with fresh parsley that has been cut into small bits.
6. Serve quickly.

Per serving: Calories: 120kcal; Fat: 7g; Carbs: 12g; Protein: 5g; Sugar: 3g

62. Lemon Herb Roasted Cauliflower

Preparation time: 10 minutes
Cooking time: 25 minutes
Servings: 4
Ingredients:

- 1 head cauliflower, cut into florets
- 2 tbsps olive oil
- Zest of 1 lemon
- 2 tbsps fresh herbs (e.g., rosemary, thyme, or parsley), cut into small bits
- Salt and pepper as needed
- Lemon wedges for presenting

Directions:

1. Warm up your oven to 425 deg.F.
2. In a bowl, blend the cauliflower florets with the olive oil, the lemon zest, the fresh herbs that have been cut into small bits, the salt, and the pepper.
3. Organize the cauliflower in a single layer on the baking sheet you have prepared.
4. Put the cauliflower in an oven that has been preheated and roast it for 20 to 25 minutes, or until it is golden brown and soft.
5. Lemon wedges should be served on a separate plate, as this is the preferred practice.

Per serving: Calories: 80kcal; Fat: 5g; Carbs: 8g; Protein: 3g; Sugar: 3g

63. Sautéed Spinach with Garlic and Lemon

Preparation time: 5 minutes
Cooking time: 5 minutes
Servings: 4

Ingredients:

- 1 lb fresh spinach, washed and trimmed
- 2 tbsps olive oil
- 3 pieces garlic, crushed
- Juice of 1 lemon
- Salt and pepper as needed

Directions:

1. Bring the olive oil to a temp. that is intermediate in your big skillet.
2. Include the garlic that has been crushed, and then sauté it for a couple of minutes until it becomes aromatic.
3. Include the fresh spinach to the skillet and toss it until it wilts, which should take around 2 to 3 minutes.
4. Drizzle the spinach with lemon juice and continue to toss until the spinach is completely included in the mixture.
5. Include salt and pepper as needed, depending on the situation.
6. Present instantly.

Per serving: Calories: 70kcal; Fat: 5g; Carbs: 4g; Protein: 3g; Sugar: 0g

64. Steamed Broccoli with Almond Slivers

Preparation time: 5 minutes
Cooking time: 5 minutes
Servings: 4
Ingredients:

- 1 lb broccoli florets
- 2 tbsps almond slivers
- 1 tbsp olive oil
- Salt and pepper as needed

- Lemon wedges for presenting (optional)

Directions:

1. Steam broccoli florets for around 5 minutes, or until they are crisp-tender.
2. Prepare the almond slivers by toasting them in a small skillet over middling temp. until they turn a light golden color.
3. Toss broccoli that has been cooked with olive oil, almond slivers that have been toasted, salt, and pepper.
4. Serve with lemon wedges, if desired on request.

Per serving: Calories: 70kcal; Fat: 5g; Carbs: 5g; Protein: 3g; Sugar: 2g

65. Oven-Roasted Zucchini and Bell Peppers

Preparation time: 10 minutes
Cooking time: 20 minutes
Servings: 4
Ingredients:

- 2 zucchini, cut
- 2 bell peppers (assorted colors), cut
- 2 tbsps olive oil
- 1 tsp dried Italian herbs
- Salt and pepper as needed
- Fresh basil for garnish (optional)

Directions:

1. Warm up your oven to 425 deg.F.
2. Blend the zucchini and bell peppers in a big bowl and toss them with olive oil, dried Italian herbs, salt, and pepper while mixing often.

3. Organize the vegetables in a single layer on the baking sheet you have prepared from using.

4. Place in an oven that has been warmed up and roast for 15 to 20 minutes, or until the edges are golden brown.

5. If desired, garnish with fresh basil after serving.

6. Serve quickly.

Per serving: Calories: 80kcal; Fat: 6g; Carbs: 7g; Protein: 2g; Sugar: 4g

66. Garlic Butter Mushrooms

Preparation time: 10 minutes
Cooking time: 10 minutes
Servings: 4
Ingredients:

- 1 lb mushrooms, cleaned and divided
- 2 tbsps unsalted butter
- 3 pieces garlic, crushed
- 1 tbsp fresh parsley, cut into small bits
- Salt and pepper as needed

Directions:

1. Melt the butter in your big skillet at a temp. that is somewhere in the middle.

2. Include the garlic that has been crushed, and then sauté it for a couple of minutes until it becomes aromatic.

3. Include mushrooms to the skillet and continue to sauté them until they release their moisture and turn a golden brown color.

4. Flavor with salt and pepper, and then sprinkle with fresh parsley that has been cut by hand.

5. After giving it a thorough stir, continue cooking for an extra 2 to 3 minutes.

6. Serve quickly.

Per serving: Calories: 80kcal; Fat: 6g; Carbs: 5g; Protein: 3g; Sugar: 2g

67. Grilled Asparagus with Balsamic Glaze

Preparation time: 10 minutes
Cooking time: 8 minutes
Servings: 4
Ingredients:

- 1 lb asparagus spears, trimmed
- 2 tbsps olive oil
- Salt and pepper as needed
- 2 tbsps balsamic glaze

Directions:

1. The grill pan should be heated to a med-high temp.

2. Put the asparagus spears in the bowl and, using olive oil, salt, and pepper, stir them together.

3. Cook the asparagus on the grill for 6 to 8 minutes, turning it occasionally, until it is soft and has a faint charred appearance.

4. Before presenting your grilled asparagus, drizzle it with a balsamic sauce; this step is optional.

5. Serve quickly.

Per serving: Calories: 70kcal; Fat: 5g; Carbs: 6g; Protein: 3g; Sugar: 3g

68. Lemon Thyme Roasted Carrots

Preparation time: 10 minutes
Cooking time: 25 minutes
Servings: 4
Ingredients:

- 1 lb carrots, that is skinned and cut into sticks
- 2 tbsps olive oil
- Zest of 1 lemon
- 1 tbsp fresh thyme leaves
- Salt and pepper as needed
- Lemon wedges for presenting (optional)

Directions:

1. Warm up your oven to 400 deg.F.
2. Put the carrot sticks in a bowl and make sure to include salt, olive oil, lemon zest, fresh thyme leaves, and pepper to the carrot sticks.
3. Organize the carrots in a single layer on the baking sheet you have prepared.
4. Roast the carrots in an oven that has been warmed up for 20 to 25 minutes, or until they are tender and have a caramelized look.
5. Lemon wedges should be served on a separate plate, as this is the preferred practice.

Per serving: Calories: 80kcal; Fat: 6g; Carbs: 7g; Protein: 1g; Sugar: 3g

69. Mashed Cauliflower with Chives

Preparation time: 10 minutes
Cooking time: 10 minutes
Servings: 4
Ingredients:

- 1 head cauliflower, cut into florets
- 2 tbsps unsalted butter
- 2 tbsps chives, cut into small bits
- Salt and pepper as needed

Directions:

1. Steam cauliflower florets for around ten minutes, or until they are very soft.
2. Put the cauliflower in a bowl once it has been drained in detail.
3. Include butter that has not been salted, cut into small bits chives, salt, and pepper to the mixture.
4. For a creamier consistency, mash the mixture until it is completely smooth using a potato masher or puree it in a blender.
5. Adjust the flavoring as needed as necessary.
6. Serve quickly.

Per serving: Calories: 80kcal; Fat: 6g; Carbs: 6g; Protein: 3g; Sugar: 3g

70. Sautéed Kale with Pine Nuts

Preparation time: 10 minutes
Cooking time: 10 minutes
Servings: 4
Ingredients:

- 1 bunch kale, stems taken out & leaves cut into small bits
- 2 tbsps olive oil
- 2 pieces garlic, crushed
- 1/4 cup pine nuts
- Salt and pepper as needed
- Lemon wedges for presenting (optional)

Directions:

1. Bring the olive oil to a temp. that is intermediate in your big skillet.
2. Include crushed garlic and pine nuts, and leave the mixture to sauté for a couple of minutes, or until the pine nuts have a mild toasty flavor.

3. Include cut into small bits kale leaves to the skillet and toss them until they are wilted and covered with oil, garlic, and pine nuts that you have added.

4. Include salt and pepper as needed, depending on the situation.

5. If necessary, squeeze lemon slices over the surface of the kale.

6. Serve quickly.

Per serving: Calories: 120kcal; Fat: 10g; Carbs: 6g; Protein: 3g; Sugar: 1g

71. Tomato Basil Caprese Salad

Preparation time: 10 minutes
Cooking time: 0 minutes
Servings: 4
Ingredients:

- 2 big tomatoes, cut
- 1 ball fresh mozzarella, cut
- Fresh basil leaves
- 2 tbsps balsamic glaze
- Salt and pepper as needed

Directions:

1. Put the slices of fresh mozzarella and tomatoes in alternate order on the serving platter you will be using.

2. Insert fresh basil leaves in between the slices of bread.

3. Apply a balsamic glaze over the salad and drizzle it over.

4. Include salt and pepper as needed, depending on the situation.

5. Serve as a refreshing salad or a side dish. This can be done instantly.

Per serving: Calories: 150kcal; Fat: 10g; Carbs: 6g; Protein: 9g; Sugar: 4g

72. Spicy Roasted Eggplant

Preparation time: 15 minutes
Cooking time: 25 minutes
Servings: 4
Ingredients:

- 1 big eggplant, cut into cubes
- 2 tbsps olive oil
- 1 tsp smoked paprika
- 1/2 tsp cayenne pepper
- 1 tsp cumin
- Salt and pepper as needed
- Fresh cilantro for garnish (optional)

Directions:

1. Warm up your oven to 425 deg.F.

2. Blend the eggplant cubes, cumin, cayenne, olive oil, smoked paprika, salt, and pepper in a bowl.

3. Spread out the flavored eggplant in a single layer on the baking sheet.

4. Roast the eggplant for 20 to 25 minutes, or until it is soft and golden brown, in your warmed up oven.

5. If necessary, garnish with fresh cilantro.

6. Present warm.

Per serving: Calories: 90kcal; Fat: 7g; Carbs: 8g; Protein: 1g; Sugar: 4g

73. Stir-Fried Cabbage and Bell Peppers

Preparation time: 10 minutes
Cooking time: 10 minutes
Servings: 4
Ingredients:

- 1/2 head cabbage, finely cut

- 2 bell peppers (assorted colors), finely cut
- 2 tbsps vegetable oil
- 1 tbsp soy sauce (low-sodium)
- 1 tsp sesame oil
- 1 tsp ginger, grated
- 2 pieces garlic, crushed
- Salt and pepper as needed
- Sesame seeds for garnish (optional)

Directions:

1. To begin, bring the vegetable oil to a med-high temp. in a wok or big skillet.
2. After including the grated ginger and smashed garlic, sauté the mixture for a minute until the aroma is released.
3. Include cabbage and bell peppers that have been finely cut into small bits to the wok and stir-fry them for 5-7 minutes, or until the veggies are crisp-tender.
4. Drizzle the vegetables with your soy sauce and sesame oil, then toss them to ensure that they are evenly coated.
5. Include salt and pepper as needed, depending on the situation.
6. If desired, garnish with toasted sesame seeds on top.
7. Serve while still hot.

Per serving: Calories: 80kcal; Fat: 5g; Carbs: 9g; Protein: 2g; Sugar: 4g

74. Greek Salad with Kalamata Olives

Preparation time: 15 minutes
Cooking time: 0 minutes
Servings: 4
Ingredients:

- 4 cups mixed salad greens
- 1 cup cherry tomatoes, divided
- 1 cucumber, cubed
- 1/2 red onion, finely cut
- 1/2 cup Kalamata olives, pitted
- 4 oz. feta cheese, crumbled
- 2 tbsps extra-virgin olive oil
- 1 tbsp red wine vinegar
- 1 tsp dried oregano
- Salt and pepper as needed

Directions:

1. First, in a big bowl, mix together the following components: mixed salad greens, cherry tomatoes, sliced cucumber, red onion that has been finely cut, Kalamata olives, and crumbled feta cheese.
2. In the small bowl you have, blend the extra-virgin olive oil, the red wine vinegar, the dried oregano, the salt, and the pepper by whisking them together.
3. Afterwards, pour the dressing over the salad and toss it until it is evenly coated.
4. Instantly present for consumption as a revitalizing Greek salad.

Per serving: Calories: 200kcal; Fat: 16g; Carbs: 10g; Protein: 6g; Sugar: 4g

75. Buttery Garlic Swiss Chard

Preparation time: 10 minutes
Cooking time: 10 minutes
Servings: 4
Ingredients:

- 1 bunch Swiss chard, stems taken out and leaves cut into small bits
- 2 tbsps unsalted butter

- 3 pieces garlic, crushed
- Salt and pepper as needed
- Lemon wedges for presenting (optional)

Directions:

1. Melt unsalted butter in a big skillet at a temp. that is close to medium.

2. Include the garlic that has been crushed, and then sauté it for a couple of minutes until it becomes aromatic.

3. Include cut into small bits Swiss chard leaves to the skillet and stir them all together until they are wilted and covered with butter and garlic powder.

4. Include salt and pepper as needed, depending on the situation.

5. In the event that it is necessary, squeeze lemon wedges over the Swiss chard.

6. Serve quickly.

Per serving: Calories: 80kcal; Fat: 6g; Carbs: 5g; Protein: 2g; Sugar: 1g

SALAD RECIPES

76. Quinoa and Avocado Salad

Preparation time: 15 minutes
Cooking time: 15 minutes
Servings: 4
Ingredients:

- 1 cup quinoa, cooked and cooled
- 1 avocado, cubed
- 1 cup cherry tomatoes, divided
- 1/2 cucumber, cubed
- 1/4 cup red onion, finely cut into small bits
- 2 tbsps fresh cilantro, cut into small bits
- 2 tbsps olive oil
- 1 tbsp lime juice
- Salt and pepper as needed

Directions:

1. Using your big bowl, mix together the quinoa that has been cooked, the cubed avocado, the cherry tomatoes, the cubed cucumber, the cut into small bits red onion, and the cut into small bits fresh cilantro.
2. In the small bowl you have, blend the lime juice and olive oil by whisking them together.
3. Pour the dressing over the salad, and then toss it until it is thoroughly blended.
4. Include salt and pepper as needed, depending on the situation.
5. Serve when chilled.

Per serving: Calories: 300kcal; Fat: 16g; Carbs: 33g; Protein: 7g; Sugar: 2g

77. Grilled Chicken Caesar Salad

Preparation time: 20 minutes
Cooking time: 15 minutes
Servings: 4
Ingredients:

- 2 boneless, skinless chicken breasts
- Salt and black pepper as needed
- 1 tbsp olive oil
- 1 head romaine lettuce, cut into small bits
- 1/2 cup cherry tomatoes, divided
- 1/4 cup Parmesan cheese, grated
- 1/4 cup Caesar dressing (low-sugar)
- Croutons for garnish (optional)

Directions:

1. Using salt and black pepper, flavor chicken breasts with salt and pepper.
2. In a grill pan, bring the olive oil to a temp. of med-high.
3. Cook your chicken breasts on the grill for 6 to 8 minutes on all sides, or until they are fully done.
4. Allow the chicken to rest for a couple of minutes, and then slice it into thin strips following this step.
5. Put the romaine lettuce, cherry tomatoes, and grilled chicken that has been sliced into pieces in the big bowl that you have.
6. Grate some Parmesan cheese and sprinkle it over the salad.
7. Afterwards, drizzle the Caesar dressing over the salad and toss it until it is evenly coated.
8. Croutons can be used as a garnish if necessary.
9. Present instantly.

Per serving: Calories: 280kcal; Fat: 15g; Carbs: 7g; Protein: 27g; Sugar: 2g

78. Spinach and Strawberry Salad

Preparation time: 15 minutes
Cooking time: 0 minutes
Servings: 4
Ingredients:

- 8 cups fresh spinach leaves, that is washed and dried
- 1 cup strawberries, hulled and cut
- 1/4 cup red onion, finely cut
- 1/4 cup feta cheese, crumbled
- 1/4 cup walnuts, cut into small bits
- 2 tbsps balsamic vinaigrette dressing (low-sugar)
- Salt and pepper as needed

Directions:

1. To begin, put the fresh spinach leaves, strawberries that have been cut into small pieces, red onion that has been finely cubed, crumbled feta cheese, and cut into small bits walnuts in a big salad bowl.
2. The second step is to drizzle the salad with balsamic vinaigrette dressing.
3. Give the salad a light gentle toss until it is evenly coated.
4. Include salt and pepper as needed, depending on the situation.
5. Present instantly.

Per serving: Calories: 150kcal; Fat: 10g; Carbs: 12g; Protein: 5g; Sugar: 5g

79. Tuna and White Bean Salad

Preparation time: 10 minutes
Servings: 4

Ingredients:

- 2 cans (15 oz each) white beans, that is drained and washed
- 2 cans (5 oz each) tuna in a water, that is drained
- 1/2 red onion, finely cut into small bits
- 1/4 cup fresh parsley, cut into small bits
- 2 tbsps capers, drained
- 2 tbsps extra-virgin olive oil
- 1 tbsp red wine vinegar
- Salt and black pepper as needed
- Lemon wedges for presenting (optional)

Directions:

1. The first step is to blend white beans, tuna that has been drained, finely sliced red onion, cut into small bits fresh parsley, and capers that have been drained in a big bowl.
2. In the small bowl you have, blend the extra-virgin olive oil and the red wine vinegar by whisking them together.
3. Afterwards, pour the dressing over the salad and toss it until it is evenly coated.
4. Salt and black pepper should be used to flavor the food as needed.
5. Serve chilled, with lemon wedges on the side, the lemon wedges being optional.

Per serving: Calories: 350kcal; Fat: 12g; Carbs: 30g; Protein: 28g; Sugar: 1g

80. Caprese Salad with Balsamic Glaze

Preparation time: 10 minutes

Cooking time: 0 minutes

Servings: 4

Ingredients:

- 4 big tomatoes, cut
- 1 ball fresh mozzarella, cut
- Fresh basil leaves
- 2 tbsps balsamic glaze
- Salt and pepper as needed

Directions:

1. Lay out your tomatoes and fresh mozzarella slices in an alternating pattern on a serving platter.
2. Insert fresh basil leaves in between the slices of bread.
3. Apply a balsamic glaze over the salad and drizzle it over.
4. Include salt and pepper as needed, depending on the situation.
5. Instantly present as a traditional Caprese salad at the table.

Per serving: Calories: 200kcal; Fat: 12g; Carbs: 12g; Protein: 12g; Sugar: 6g

81. Roasted Beet Salad with Goat Cheese

Preparation time: 15 minutes

Cooking time: 45 minutes (for roasting beets)

Servings: 4

Ingredients:

- 4 medium beets, roasted, skinned, and cubed
- 4 cups mixed salad greens
- 1/2 cup goat cheese, crumbled
- 1/4 cup walnuts, cut into small bits
- 2 tbsps balsamic vinaigrette dressing (low-sugar)

- Salt and black pepper as needed

Directions:

1. Warm up your oven to 400 deg.F. Wrap beets in foil and roast them for 45 minutes, or until they are soft. After they have cooled, skin and dice them.
2. Using a big bowl, mix together the beets that have been roasted and cubed, the mixed salad greens, the crumbled goat cheese, and the cut into small bits walnuts.
3. The third step is to drizzle the salad with balsamic vinaigrette dressing.
4. Give the salad a light toss as long as it is evenly coated.
5. The dish should be flavored with salt and black pepper as needed.
6. Serve when chilled.

Per serving: Calories: 250kcal; Fat: 15g; Carbs: 23g; Protein: 8g; Sugar: 10g

82. Shrimp and Avocado Salad

Preparation time: 20 minutes

Cooking time: 5 minutes

Servings: 4

Ingredients:

- 1 lb shrimp, skinned and deveined
- 1 tbsp olive oil
- Salt and black pepper as needed
- 8 cups mixed salad greens
- 2 avocados, cubed
- 1 cup cherry tomatoes, divided
- 1/4 cup red onion, finely cut
- 2 tbsps cilantro, cut into small bits
- 2 tbsps lime juice
- 1 tbsp olive oil

Directions:

1. To begin, bring the olive oil to a temp. of med-high in your skillet.
2. Include salt and black pepper to the shrimp, and then sauté them in the skillet for 3 to 5 minutes, or until they are completely cooked through.
3. In a big bowl, include the following components: mixed salad greens, cut into small bits avocados, cherry tomatoes, red onion that has been finely cut, and shrimp that has been cooked.
4. In the small bowl you have, blend the olive oil and lime juice by whisking them together.
5. The fifth step is to pour the dressing over the salad and then gently toss it until it is completely blended.
6. Put cut into small bits cilantro on top as a garnish.
7. Present instantly.

Per serving: Calories: 320kcal; Fat: 20g; Carbs: 18g; Protein: 22g; Sugar: 3g

83. Avocado and Tomato Salad with Lime Dressing

Preparation time: 10 minutes
Cooking time: 0 minutes
Servings: 4
Ingredients:

- 2 avocados, cubed
- 2 cups cherry tomatoes, divided
- 1/4 cup red onion, finely cut into small bits
- 2 tbsps fresh cilantro, cut into small bits
- 2 tbsps lime juice

- 2 tbsps olive oil
- Salt and pepper as needed

Directions:

1. In a big bowl, include the following components: cubed avocados, cherry tomatoes that have been separated, cut into small bits red onion, and cut into small bits fresh cilantro.
2. Put the lime juice, olive oil, salt, and pepper in a small bowl and whisk them together until they are combined.
3. Pour the dressing over the salad, then carefully toss it until it is evenly coated with the dressing.
4. Present instantly.

Per serving: Calories: 200kcal; Fat: 16g; Carbs: 15g; Protein: 2g; Sugar: 3g

84. Kale and Quinoa Salad with Lemon Vinaigrette

Preparation time: 20 minutes
Cooking time: 15 minutes
Servings: 4
Ingredients:

- 1 cup quinoa, cooked and cooled
- 4 cups kale, stems taken out & leaves cut into small bits
- 1 cup cherry tomatoes, divided
- 1/4 cup feta cheese, crumbled
- 1/4 cup pine nuts, toasted
- 2 tbsps olive oil
- 2 tbsps lemon juice
- 1 tsp Dijon mustard
- Salt and pepper as needed

Directions:

1. In a big bowl, include quinoa that has been cooked, cut into small bits kale,

the cherry tomatoes that have been separated, crumbled feta cheese, and pine nuts that have been toasted.

2. The second step is to blend the olive oil, lemon juice, Dijon mustard, salt, and pepper in a small bowl and mix them together.

3. Pour the dressing over the salad, then carefully toss it until it is evenly coated with the dressing.

4. Pour cold and serve.

Per serving: Calories: 320kcal; Fat: 18g; Carbs: 32g; Protein: 9g; Sugar: 3g

85. Cucumber and Radish Salad

Preparation time: 10 minutes

Cooking time: 0 minutes

Servings: 4

Ingredients:

- 2 cucumbers, finely cut
- 1 bunch radishes, finely cut
- 1/4 cup red onion, finely cut
- 2 tbsps fresh dill, cut into small bits
- 2 tbsps white wine vinegar
- 1 tbsp olive oil
- Salt and pepper as needed

Directions:

1. To begin, blend the cucumbers, radishes, red onion, and fresh dill that have been finely cut into small bits in a big bowl.

2. The second step is to blend the white wine vinegar, olive oil, salt, and pepper in a small basin and mix them together.

3. Pour the dressing over the salad, then gently toss it until it is evenly coated with the dressing.

4. Pour cold and serve.

Per serving: Calories: 80kcal; Fat: 5g; Carbs: 10g; Protein: 2g; Sugar: 4g

86. Watermelon and Feta Salad

Preparation time: 15 minutes

Cooking time: 0 minutes

Servings: 4

Ingredients:

- 4 cups watermelon, cubed
- 1 cup feta cheese, crumbled
- 1/4 cup fresh mint leaves, cut into small bits
- 2 tbsps balsamic reduction
- Salt as needed
- Black pepper as needed

Directions:

1. In a big bowl, include watermelon that has been cubed, feta cheese that has been crumbled, and fresh mint leaves that have been cut.

2. Pour the balsamic reduction over the salad and taste it.

3. Give the salad a light gentle toss until it is evenly coated.

4. Salt and black pepper should be used to flavor the food as needed.

5. Serve when chilled.

Per serving: Calories: 180kcal; Fat: 8g; Carbs: 24g; Protein: 6g; Sugar: 18g

87. Broccoli and Cranberry Salad

Preparation time: 15 minutes

Cooking time: 0 minutes

Servings: 4

Ingredients:

- 4 cups broccoli florets, blanched and cooled
- 1/2 cup dried cranberries
- 1/4 cup red onion, finely cut into small bits
- 1/4 cup sunflower seeds
- 1/2 cup Greek yogurt (plain, non-fat)
- 2 tbsps apple cider vinegar
- 1 tbsp honey or a sugar substitute
- Salt and pepper as needed

Directions:

1. To begin, blend broccoli florets that have been blanched, dried cranberries, sliced red onion, and sunflower seeds in a big bowl before proceeding.
2. In a small bowl, blend the Greek yogurt, apple cider vinegar, honey (or sugar replacement), salt, and pepper by whisking them together.
3. Afterwards, pour the dressing over the salad and toss it until it is evenly coated.
4. Pour cold and serve.

Per serving: Calories: 160kcal; Fat: 7g; Carbs: 23g; Protein: 7g; Sugar: 12g

88. Chicken and Apple Salad with Walnuts

Preparation time: 20 minutes
Cooking time: 10 minutes
Servings: 4
Ingredients:

- 2 boneless, skinless chicken breasts
- Salt and black pepper as needed
- 1 tbsp olive oil
- 4 cups mixed salad greens

- 2 apples, cored and cut
- 1/2 cup walnuts, cut into small bits
- 1/4 cup blue cheese, crumbled
- 2 tbsps balsamic vinaigrette dressing (low-sugar)

Directions:

1. Using salt and black pepper, flavor chicken breasts with salt and pepper.
2. In your skillet, bring the olive oil to a temp. of medium-high.
3. Cook your chicken breasts on the grill for 5 to 7 minutes on all sides, or until they are fully done.
4. Allow the chicken to rest for a couple of minutes, and then slice it into thin strips following this step.
5. In a big bowl, include several different types of salad greens, grilled chicken that has been cut into pieces, cut into small bits walnuts, cubed apples, and crumbled blue cheese.
6. Balsamic vinaigrette dressing should be drizzled over the salad at this point.
7. Carefully toss until everything is completely blended.
8. Present instantly.

Per serving: Calories: 340kcal; Fat: 20g; Carbs: 24g; Protein: 22g; Sugar: 16g

89. Mango and Black Bean Salad

Preparation time: 15 minutes
Cooking time: 0 minutes
Servings: 4
Ingredients:

- 2 mangos, cubed

- 1 tin (15 oz) black beans, that is drained and washed
- 1 red bell pepper, cubed
- 1/4 cup red onion, finely cut into small bits
- 1/4 cup fresh cilantro, cut into small bits
- 2 tbsps lime juice
- 2 tbsps olive oil
- Salt and pepper as needed

Directions:

1. In a big bowl, include the following components: cubed mangoes, black beans that have been drained, cubed red bell pepper, sliced red onion, and cut into small bits fresh cilantro.
2. Put the lime juice, olive oil, salt, and pepper in a small bowl and whisk them together until they are combined.
3. Pour the dressing over the salad, then gently toss it until it is evenly coated with the dressing.
4. Pour cold and serve.

Per serving: Calories: 260kcal; Fat: 8g; Carbs: 42g; Protein: 8g; Sugar: 20g

90. Waldorf Salad with Greek Yogurt Dressing

Preparation time: 15 minutes

Cooking time: 0 minutes

Servings: 4

Ingredients:

- 2 apples, cored and cubed
- 1 cup celery, finely cut
- 1 cup grapes, divided
- 1/2 cup walnuts, cut into small bits

- 1/2 cup Greek yogurt (plain, non-fat)
- 1 tbsp honey or a sugar substitute
- 1 tsp lemon juice
- Salt as needed

Directions:

1. Put the cubed apples, celery that has been finely cut, grapes that have been separated, and walnuts that have been cut into small bits into the big bowl.
2. In a small bowl, blend Greek yogurt, honey (or sugar replacement), lemon juice, and a slight amount of salt by whisking the entire components together.
3. Pour the dressing over the salad, then gently toss it until it is evenly coated with the dressing.
4. Pour cold and serve.

Per serving: Calories: 220kcal; Fat: 10g; Carbs: 32g; Protein: 6g; Sugar: 24g

MEAT RECIPES

91. Herbed Grilled Pork Chops

Preparation time: 10 minutes

Cooking time: 15 minutes

Servings: 4

Ingredients:

- 4 pork chops
- 2 tbsps olive oil
- 1 tbsp fresh rosemary, cut into small bits
- 1 tbsp fresh thyme, cut into small bits
- 1 tsp garlic powder
- Salt and black pepper as needed

Directions:

1. Bring the temp. of the grill up to a med-high level.
2. In a bowl, blend the following components: garlic powder, salt, black pepper, cut into small bits fresh rosemary, and cut into small bits fresh thyme; olive oil; and both of these ingredients.
3. Coat each pork chop with the herb mixture using a scrub brush.
4. Cook pork chops on the grill for 6 to 8 minutes on all sides, or until they reach an internal temp. of 145 deg.F.
5. The pork chops should be allowed to rest for a couple of minutes before being presented to the audience.

Per serving: Calories: 250kcal; Fat: 14g; Carbs: 0g; Protein: 30g; Sugar: 0g

92. Rosemary Roasted Lamb Chops

Preparation time: 15 minutes (plus marinating time)

Cooking time: 20 minutes

Servings: 4

Ingredients:

- 8 lamb chops
- 2 tbsps olive oil
- 2 tbsps fresh rosemary, cut into small bits
- 3 pieces garlic, crushed
- Salt and pepper as needed

Directions:

1. The first step is to blend the following components in a bowl: olive oil, cut into small bits rosemary, crushed garlic, salt, and pepper.
2. To ensure that the lamb chops are evenly coated with the rosemary mixture, put them in a plate and massage it over them by hand.
3. Put the marinade in the fridge for close to an hour.
4. Warm up your oven to 400 deg.F.
5. Put the lamb chops that have been marinated on the baking sheet.
6. The sixth step is to roast the meat for nearly twenty minutes, or until the internal temp. reaches the level of doneness that you want.
7. When it comes time to offer the lamb chops, give them a couple of minutes to rest before doing so.

Per serving: Calories: 350kcal; Fat: 25g; Carbs: 0g; Protein: 30g; Sugar: 0g

93. Grilled Lemon Herb Pork Chops

Preparation time: 15 minutes (plus marinating time)

Cooking time: 15 minutes

Servings: 4

Ingredients:

- 4 boneless pork chops
- Zest and juice of 1 lemon
- 2 tbsps olive oil
- 2 pieces garlic, crushed
- 1 tsp dried oregano
- 1 tsp dried thyme
- Salt and pepper as needed

Directions:

1. In a small bowl, blend the lemon zest, lemon juice, olive oil, crushed garlic, dried oregano, dried thyme, salt, and pepper by whisking the entire components together.
2. Following the placement of the pork chops in the shallow dish, pour the marinade over the pork chops. Take care that the chops are adequately covered.
3. Put the marinade in the fridge for close to half an hour.
4. Bring the temp. of the grill up to a medium-high level.
5. Cook pork chops on the grill for around 6 to 8 minutes on all sides, or until they are completely cooked through.
6. In order to prepare the chops for presentation, you should give them a couple of minutes to rest.

Per serving: Calories: 250kcal; Fat: 15g; Carbs: 1g; Protein: 26g; Sugar: 0g

94. Herb-Roasted Pork Tenderloin

Preparation time: 10 minutes (plus marinating time)

Cooking time: 25 minutes

Servings: 4

Ingredients:

- 1 pork tenderloin (about 1 lb)
- 2 tbsps olive oil
- 2 pieces garlic, crushed
- 1 tsp dried rosemary
- 1 tsp dried thyme
- Salt and pepper as needed

Directions:

1. In a small bowl, blend the following components: olive oil, smashed garlic, dried rosemary, dried thyme, salt, and pepper by mixing them together.
2. Put the pork tenderloin in a dish and spread the herb mixture all over it, making sure that it is evenly distributed.
3. Marinate the meat in the fridge for close to an hour or overnight.
4. Warm up your oven to 400 deg.F.
5. Put the pork tenderloin that has been marinated on the baking sheet that you have.
6. Roast for almost 25 minutes, or until the temp. on the inside reaches 145 deg.F.
7. Before cutting the pork, allow it to rest for a couple of minutes before beginning to cut it.

Per serving: Calories: 220kcal; Fat: 12g; Carbs: 1g; Protein: 26g; Sugar: 0g

95. Garlic and Herb Marinated Beef Kebabs

Preparation time: 20 minutes (plus marinating time)

Cooking time: 10 minutes

Servings: 4

Ingredients:

- 1 lb beef sirloin or tenderloin, cut into cubes
- 1/4 cup olive oil
- 4 pieces garlic, crushed
- 2 tbsps fresh parsley, cut into small bits
- 1 tsp dried oregano
- 1 tsp dried thyme
- Salt and pepper as needed
- Bell peppers, onions, and cherry tomatoes for skewering

Directions:

1. In a dish, mix together olive oil, salt, pepper, dried oregano, dried thyme, cut into small bits parsley, and crushed garlic.
2. Include the beef cubes to the marinade, being sure to coat them completely. Soak for one hour in the fridge.
3. Set the grill's temp. to medium-high.
4. Thread cherry tomatoes, bell peppers, onions, and marinated meat cubes onto skewers.
5. Cook the kebabs for 8 to 10 minutes, rotating them occasionally, or until the beef is cooked to your preference.
6. Accompany hot with your preferred side dishes.

Per serving: Calories: 280kcal; Fat: 20g; Carbs: 5g; Protein: 22g; Sugar: 2g

96. Stuffed Bell Peppers with Lean Ground Beef

Preparation time: 20 minutes

Cooking time: 35 minutes

Servings: 4

Ingredients:

- 4 bell peppers, divided and seeds taken out
- 1 lb lean ground beef
- 1 onion, cubed
- 2 pieces garlic, crushed
- 1 cup quinoa, cooked
- 1 tin (14 oz) cubed tomatoes, drained
- 1 tsp dried oregano
- 1 tsp ground cumin
- Salt and pepper as needed
- 1 cup shredded mozzarella cheese

Directions:

1. Warm up your oven to 375 deg.F.
2. Brown the ground beef at a med-high temp. in your skillet.
3. Include the smashed garlic and cut into small bits onion. Cook until the onion becomes clear.
4. Put cooked ground beef, cooked quinoa, cut into small bits tomatoes, ground cumin, dried oregano, salt, and pepper in a big bowl.
5. Stuff your ground beef mixture into each half of a bell pepper.
6. Transfer the filled bell peppers to the baking dish. Top with mozzarella cheese that has been shredded.
7. Bake for 30 to 35 minutes, or until the cheese is bubbling and melted and the peppers are soft.
8. Present warm.

Per serving: Calories: 400kcal; Fat: 15g; Carbs: 35g; Protein: 30g; Sugar: 7g

97. Zesty Baked Beef Thighs

Preparation time: 15 minutes (plus marinating time)

Cooking time: 30 minutes

Servings: 4

Ingredients:

- 4 bone-in, skinless beef thighs
- 2 tbsps olive oil
- 2 pieces garlic, crushed
- 1 tsp paprika
- 1 tsp cumin
- 1 tsp chili powder
- Salt and pepper as needed
- Fresh cilantro for garnish (optional)

Directions:

1. Blend the olive oil, crushed garlic, paprika, cumin, chili powder, salt, and pepper in a small bowl.
2. Transfer the beef thighs to a platter and evenly coat them with the flavorful mixture.
3. Marinate for about half an hour in the fridge.
4. Warm up your oven to 375 deg.F.
5. Organize the beef thighs marinated on your baking sheet.
6. Bake for around 30 minutes, or until 165 deg.F is reached internally.
7. If necessary, garnish with fresh cilantro prior to presenting.

Per serving: Calories: 300kcal; Fat: 20g; Carbs: 1g; Protein: 28g; Sugar: 0g

98. Mushroom and Spinach Stuffed Pork Tenderloin

Preparation time: 20 minutes

Cooking time: 30 minutes

Servings: 4

Ingredients:

- 1 pork tenderloin (about 1 lb)
- 1 cup baby spinach, cut into small bits
- 1 cup mushrooms, finely cut into small bits
- 2 pieces garlic, crushed
- 1 tbsp olive oil
- Salt and pepper as needed
- Cooking twine

Directions:

1. Warm up your oven to 375 deg.F.
2. Warm the olive oil in your skillet to a middling temp. Include the crushed garlic and sauté it until aromatic.
3. Include cut into small bits spinach and mushrooms to your skillet. Cook until the liquid has gone and the vegetables are tender. Include pepper and salt for flavoring.
4. Slice the pork tenderloin in half lengthwise and open it up like a book to create a butterfly effect.
5. Transfer the mixture of mushrooms and spinach to one side of the pork belly.
6. Fold the pork's other side over the filling and tie it off with cooking twine.
7. Transfer the filled pork tenderloin to a baking sheet and bake it for about half an hour, or until the internal temp. reaches 145 deg.F.
8. Rest the pork prior to cutting and serving.

Per serving: Calories: 240kcal; Fat: 10g; Carbs: 3g; Protein: 34g; Sugar: 1g

99. Vegetable and Ground Beef Skillet

Preparation time: 15 minutes
Cooking time: 20 minutes
Servings: 4
Ingredients:

- 1 lb lean ground beef
- 1 onion, cubed
- 2 bell peppers, cut
- 2 zucchinis, cut
- 2 tomatoes, cubed
- 2 pieces garlic, crushed
- 1 tsp Italian flavoring
- Salt and pepper as needed
- Fresh parsley for garnish (optional)

Directions:

1. Brown the ground beef at a med-high temp. in a big skillet.
2. Include the smashed garlic and cut into small bits onion. Cook until the onion becomes clear.
3. Include cubed tomatoes, cut into small bits bell peppers, and zucchini to the skillet. Mix thoroughly.
4. Include salt, pepper, and Italian flavoring to the dish. Simmer until the veggies are soft and the flavors blend.
5. If necessary, garnish with fresh parsley prior to presenting.

Per serving: Calories: 280kcal; Fat: 15g; Carbs: 10g; Protein: 25g; Sugar: 6g

100. Balsamic Glazed Pork Chops

Preparation time: 10 minutes (plus marinating time)
Cooking time: 20 minutes
Servings: 4
Ingredients:

- 4 boneless pork chops
- 1/4 cup balsamic vinegar
- 2 tbsps olive oil
- 2 tbsps Dijon mustard
- 2 pieces garlic, crushed
- 1 tbsp honey
- Salt and pepper as needed
- Fresh rosemary for garnish (optional)

Directions:

1. Blend the olive oil, Dijon mustard, honey, smashed garlic, balsamic vinegar, salt, and pepper in a bowl.
2. Transfer the pork chops to a platter and cover with the balsamic glaze. Make sure the chops have a good coating.
3. Marinate for nearly an hour in the fridge.
4. Warm up your skillet or grill to a medium-high temp.
5. Cook the pork chops for about 8 to 10 minutes on all sides, or until they are cooked through, on a grill or pan.
6. If necessary, garnish with fresh rosemary prior to presenting.

Per serving: Calories: 280kcal; Fat: 15g; Carbs: 8g; Protein: 25g; Sugar: 6g

101. Beef and Vegetable Stir-Fry

Preparation time: 15 minutes
Cooking time: 10 minutes

Servings: 4

Ingredients:

- 1 lb lean beef strips
- 2 cups broccoli florets
- 1 bell pepper, finely cut
- 1 carrot, julienned
- 2 tbsps low-sodium soy sauce
- 1 tbsp olive oil
- 2 pieces garlic, crushed
- 1 tsp ginger, grated
- 1 tbsp sesame seeds (optional)
- Green onions for garnish (optional)

Directions:

1. To begin, bring the olive oil to a med-high temp. in a wok or big skillet.
2. Incorporate grated ginger and crushed garlic, and continue to sauté for a couple of minutes.
3. Stir-frying the beef strips until they are browned.
4. Incorporate carrots, bell peppers, and broccoli into the dish. Stir-frying should be continued for a further 5 to 7 minutes until the vegetables are crisp-tender.
5. After pouring the soy sauce over the stir-fry, toss it to ensure that it is evenly coated.
6. To finish, sprinkle with toasted sesame seeds and, if desired, garnish with cut into small bits green onions.
7. Present instantly.

Per serving: Calories: 280kcal; Fat: 14g; Carbs: 9g; Protein: 30g; Sugar: 3g

102. Greek Salad with Grilled Lamb

Preparation time: 20 minutes (plus marinating time)

Cooking time: 15 minutes

Servings: 4

Ingredients:

- 1 lb lamb chops
- 1 lemon, juiced
- 2 tbsps olive oil
- 3 pieces garlic, crushed
- 1 tsp dried oregano
- Salt and pepper as needed
- 4 cups mixed salad greens
- 1 cucumber, cut
- 1 cup cherry tomatoes, divided
- 1/2 cup Kalamata olives
- 1/2 cup feta cheese, crumbled

Directions:

1. Pour the salt, lemon juice, olive oil, crushed garlic, dried oregano, and pepper into your bowl and mix them together until they are combined.
2. After placing the lamb chops on a plate, pour the marinade over them and put them away. Take care that the chops are adequately covered.
3. Put the marinade in the fridge for close to 2 hours.
4. Bring the temp. of the grill up to a medium-high level.
5. Put the lamb chops on the grill and cook them for around 6 to 8 minutes on all sides, or until they reach the desired level of doneness.
6. In a big salad bowl, blend the following components: feta cheese, cherry

tomatoes, cucumbers that have been cut into cubes, and mixed greens.

7. Organize lamb chops that have been grilled on top of the salad.

8. Present instantly.

Per serving: Calories: 400kcal; Fat: 28g; Carbs: 10g; Protein: 30g; Sugar: 4g

103. Spinach and Mushroom Stuffed Beef Rolls

Preparation time: 25 minutes
Cooking time: 25 minutes
Servings: 4
Ingredients:

- 4 thin beef sirloin or flank steak slices
- 2 cups fresh spinach, cut into small bits
- 1 cup mushrooms, finely cut into small bits
- 2 pieces garlic, crushed
- 1/2 cup low-fat mozzarella cheese, shredded
- 2 tbsps olive oil
- Salt and pepper as needed
- Toothpicks or kitchen twine for securing rolls

Directions:

1. Warm up your oven to 375 deg.F.

2. Bring the olive oil to a temp. that is on the middle in your skillet. If you want to include crushed garlic, sauté it until it becomes aromatic.

3. After the entire liquid has evaporated, include the cut into small bits mushrooms and continue to cook. Include cut into small bits spinach, then continue cooking until it has

wilted. Salt and pepper should be used to flavor.

4. Organize the beef slices in a single layer and then distribute the spinach and mushroom mixture evenly across the beef slices.

5. Sprinkle shredded mozzarella cheese on top of each sliced cheese.

6. Toothpicks or kitchen twine can be used to secure the beef slices after they have been rolled up.

7. Warm the olive oil in a skillet that can go in the oven to a medium-high temp.

8. Once the meat rolls have been cooked on all sides, sear them.

9. Put the skillet in the oven that has been preheated, and bake it for 20 to 25 minutes, or until the meat is completely cooked through.

10. Before cutting the rolls and serving them, allow them to rest for a couple of minutes prior to doing so.

Per serving: Calories: 320kcal; Fat: 22g; Carbs: 3g; Protein: 28g; Sugar: 1g

104. Garlic and Rosemary Roasted Pork Tenderloin

Preparation time: 10 minutes
Cooking time: 25 minutes
Servings: 4

Ingredients:

- 1 lb pork tenderloin
- 2 tbsps olive oil
- 3 pieces garlic, crushed
- 1 tbsp fresh rosemary, cut into small bits
- 1 tsp Dijon mustard

- Salt and black pepper as needed

Directions:

1. Warm up your oven to 400 deg.F.
2. In the small bowl you have, blend the following components: olive oil, garlic that has been smashed, fresh rosemary that has been cut into small bits, Dijon mustard, salt, and black pepper.
3. The third step is to rub the pork tenderloin with the mixture of garlic and rosemary. Let it sit in the marinade for close to half an hour.
4. Put the pork tenderloin that has been marinated on a roasting pan.
5. Roast for 25 minutes, or until the temp. on the inside reaches 145 deg.F.
6. Before chopping the pork, let it to rest for a couple of minutes with the lid turned down.

Per serving: Calories: 220kcal; Fat: 10g; Carbs: 1g; Protein: 30g; Sugar: 0g

105. Citrus-Marinated Grilled Steak

Preparation time: 15 minutes (plus marinating time)

Cooking time: 15 minutes

Servings: 4

Ingredients:

- 1 lb sirloin or flank steak
- 1 orange, juiced
- 1 lime, juiced
- 2 tbsps soy sauce (low-sodium)
- 2 tbsps olive oil
- 2 pieces garlic, crushed
- 1 tsp ground cumin
- Salt and pepper as needed

- Fresh cilantro for garnish (optional)

Directions:

1. First, in a bowl, blend the following components: orange juice, lime juice, soy sauce, olive oil, crushed garlic, ground cumin, salt, and pepper. Whisk the entire components together.
2. After placing the steak in a dish, pour the citrus marinade over it and set it aside. Check to see that the meat is evenly coated.
3. Put the marinade in the fridge for close to two hours.
4. Bring the temp. of the grill up to a medium-high level.
5. Put the steak on the grill and cook it for around 6 to 8 minutes on all sides, or until it reaches the desired level of doneness.
6. Prior to cutting the steak, allow it to rest for a couple of minutes beforehand.
7. In the event that it is required, garnish with fresh cilantro and then present.

Per serving: Calories: 300kcal; Fat: 15g; Carbs: 5g; Protein: 35g; Sugar: 2g

FISH RECIPES

106. Garlic Butter Shrimp and Broccoli

Preparation time: 10 minutes
Cooking time: 15 minutes
Servings: 4
Ingredients:

- 1 lb big shrimp, skinned and deveined
- 2 tbsps unsalted butter
- 4 pieces garlic, crushed
- 1 tsp red pepper flakes
- 1 lb broccoli florets
- Salt and black pepper as needed
- Lemon wedges for presenting

Directions:

1. Melt the butter in your big skillet at a temp. that is somewhere in the middle.
2. Include smashed garlic and crushed red pepper flakes to the mixture. Sauté for a couple of minutes till the aroma is released.
3. Include shrimp to the skillet and cook them for 3 to 4 minutes, or until they turn pink.
4. After adding broccoli florets to the skillet, continue to sauté the broccoli for an extra 5 to 7 minutes, or until it reaches a crisp-tender consistency.
5. Flavor with salt and black pepper.
6. It is advised that lemon wedges be served on a separate plate after the main course.

Per serving: Calories: 180kcal; Fat: 8g; Carbs: 8g; Protein: 20g; Sugar: 2g

107. Spicy Cajun Grilled Catfish

Preparation time: 10 minutes
Cooking time: 10 minutes
Servings: 4
Ingredients:

- 4 catfish fillets
- 2 tbsps olive oil
- 1 tbsp Cajun flavoring
- 1 tsp smoked paprika
- 1/2 tsp garlic powder
- 1/2 tsp onion powder
- 1/4 tsp cayenne pepper (adjust as needed)
- Lemon wedges for presenting

Directions:

1. Bring the temp. of the grill up to a med-high level.
2. Coat both sides of the catfish fillets with olive oil and brush them out.
3. In your bowl, blend the following components: garlic powder, onion powder, Cajun flavoring, smoked paprika, and cayenne pepper for a complete mixture.
4. Make sure that the spice combination is evenly distributed on both sides of each catfish fillet.
5. Cook the catfish on the grill for 4 to 5 minutes on all sides, or until it crumbles easily when tested with a fork.
6. It is advised that lemon wedges be served on a separate plate after the main course.

Per serving: Calories: 220kcal; Fat: 12g; Carbs: 1g; Protein: 25g; Sugar: 0g

108. Almond-Crusted Baked Snapper

Preparation time: 15 minutes
Cooking time: 15 minutes
Servings: 4.
Ingredients:

- 4 snapper fillets
- 1/2 cup almonds, finely cut into small bits
- 1/4 cup whole wheat breadcrumbs
- 1 tsp dried oregano
- 1 tsp garlic powder
- 2 tbsps Dijon mustard
- 1 tbsp olive oil
- Lemon wedges for presenting

Directions:

1. Warm up your oven to 400 deg.F.
2. Almonds that have been cut into small bits, breadcrumbs, dried oregano, and garlic powder should be mixed together in a shallow dish.
3. To prepare the snapper fillets, first brush them with Dijon mustard, and then coat them with the almond mixture.
4. Put the fillets on a baking sheet that has been lined with parchment paper.
5. Olive oil should be drizzled over the top of each fillet.
6. Put the snapper in the oven and bake for 15 minutes, or until the snapper is fully cooked and the crust is golden brown.
7. Lemon wedges should be served on a separate plate, as this is the preferred practice.

Per serving: Calories: 250kcal; Fat: 14g; Carbs: 7g; Protein: 25g; Sugar: 1g

109. Teriyaki Glazed Tilapia

Preparation time: 10 minutes
Cooking time: 15 minutes
Servings: 4
Ingredients:

- 4 tilapia fillets
- 1/4 cup low-sodium soy sauce
- 2 tbsps honey or a sugar substitute
- 1 tbsp rice vinegar
- 1 tsp grated ginger
- 2 pieces garlic, crushed
- 1 tbsp sesame seeds for garnish
- Sliced green onions for garnish

Directions:

1. Warm up your oven to 400 deg.F.
2. In a bowl, blend your soy sauce, honey (or sugar equivalent), rice vinegar, grated ginger, and smashed garlic. Mix the entire ingredients simultaneously.
3. Put the tilapia fillets in the baking dish, and then pour the teriyaki sauce over them.
4. Bake the tilapia for 15 minutes, or until it reaches the desired level of doneness.
5. Prior to presentation, garnish with green onions and sesame seeds that have been cut into small bits into chunks.

Per serving: Calories: 180kcal; Fat: 3.5g; Carbs: 9g; Protein: 25g; Sugar: 6g

110. Blackened Tilapia Tacos with Cabbage Slaw

Preparation time: 15 minutes
Cooking time: 10 minutes
Servings: 4

Ingredients:

- 4 tilapia fillets
- 2 tsps blackened flavoring
- 1 tbsp olive oil
- 8 small whole wheat tortillas
- 2 cups shredded cabbage
- 1/2 cup Greek yogurt
- 1 tbsp lime juice
- Fresh cilantro for garnish

Directions:

1. Smear tilapia fillets with a spice that has been blackened.
2. In your skillet, bring the olive oil to a temp. of med-high.
3. The tilapia should be cooked for 3 to 4 minutes on all sides, or until it can be easily flaked with a fork.
4. To make the slaw, blend the shredded cabbage, Greek yogurt, and lime juice in the bowl you have available to you.
5. Warm the tortillas in your microwave or dry skillet.
6. Prepare tacos by adding fish on each tortilla and topping them with cabbage slaw.
7. The presentation should be finished with a garnish of fresh cilantro.

Per serving: Calories: 250kcal; Fat: 7g; Carbs: 25g; Protein: 22g; Sugar: 3g

111. Pan-Seared Lemon Garlic Scallops

Preparation time: 10 minutes
Cooking time: 5 minutes
Servings: 4
Ingredients:

- 1 lb big sea scallops

- 2 tbsps olive oil
- 3 pieces garlic, crushed
- Zest and juice of 1 lemon
- 2 tbsps fresh parsley, cut into small bits
- Salt and black pepper as needed
- Lemon wedges for presenting

Directions:

1. When the scallops are completely dry, pat them dry using paper towels and then flavor them with salt and black pepper.
2. In your big skillet, bring the olive oil to a temp. of medium-high.
3. Include scallops to the skillet and sear them for 2 to 3 minutes on all sides, or until they have a golden brown color altogether.
4. Include crushed garlic to your skillet and sauté it for a couple of minutes until it achieves a pleasant aroma.
5. Sprinkle the scallops with cut into small bits fresh parsley and lemon zest, then drizzle lemon juice over the scallops.
6. Present the dish in a heated state, with lemon wedges on the side.

Per serving: Calories: 150kcal; Fat: 7g; Carbs: 4g; Protein: 18g; Sugar: 0g

112. Herb-Crusted Baked Halibut

Preparation time: 15 minutes
Cooking time: 20 minutes
Servings: 4
Ingredients:

- 4 halibut fillets
- 2 tbsps olive oil
- 2 tbsps fresh parsley, cut into small bits

- 1 tbsp fresh thyme, cut into small bits
- 1 tbsp fresh rosemary, cut into small bits
- 1 tsp garlic powder
- Salt and black pepper as needed
- Lemon wedges for presenting

Directions:

1. Warm up your oven to 400 deg.F.
2. On a baking sheet that has been lined with parchment paper, arrange the halibut fillets in a single layer.
3. Blend the following components in a bowl: olive oil, cut into small bits fresh parsley, cut into small bits fresh thyme, cut into small bits fresh rosemary, garlic powder, salt, and black pepper. Mix each of these ingredients.
4. Apply a little coating of the herb mixture to each fillet of halibut.
5. Put the halibut in the oven and bake for 20 minutes or until it is completely cooked through.
6. It is advised that lemon wedges be served on a separate plate after the main course.

Per serving: Calories: 230kcal; Fat: 12g; Carbs: 0g; Protein: 30g; Sugar: 0g

113. Coconut Lime Shrimp Stir-Fry

Preparation time: 15 minutes

Cooking time: 10 minutes

Servings: 4

Ingredients:

- 1 lb big shrimp, skinned and deveined
- 2 tbsps coconut oil
- 1 bell pepper, finely cut

- 1 cup snow peas, ends trimmed
- 1 carrot, julienned
- Zest and juice of 2 limes
- 2 tbsps low-sodium soy sauce
- 1 tbsp fish sauce
- 1 tsp honey or a sugar substitute
- Fresh cilantro for garnish

Directions:

1. Bring the coconut oil to a med-high temp. in your wok or big skillet.
2. After adding the shrimp, stir-fry them for 2 to 3 minutes, or until they turn pink. First, remove the shrimp from the wok, and then put them away.
3. Put the carrot, snow peas, and bell pepper into the same skillet that you used earlier. To ensure that the vegetables are crisp-tender, stir-fry them for 3 to 4 minutes.
4. Put the shrimp that have been cooked back into the wok.
5. In a small bowl, blend the lime zest, lime juice, soy sauce, fish sauce, and honey by whisking them together. Apply the sauce to the shrimp and veggies and put them away.
6. Blend the entire ingredients and toss so they are evenly coated and heated thoroughly.
7. Garnish using fresh cilantro prior to presenting.

Per serving: Calories: 220kcal; Fat: 10g; Carbs: 10g; Protein: 22g; Sugar: 4g

114. Pistachio-Crusted Salmon

Preparation time: 15 minutes

Cooking time: 15 minutes

Servings: 4

Ingredients:

- 4 salmon fillets
- 1/2 cup pistachios, finely cut into small bits
- 1/4 cup whole wheat breadcrumbs
- 1 tsp dried thyme
- 1 tsp garlic powder
- 2 tbsps Dijon mustard
- 1 tbsp olive oil
- Lemon wedges for presenting

Directions:

1. Warm up your oven to 400 deg.F.
2. Blend cut into small bits pistachios, breadcrumbs, dried thyme, and garlic powder in a plate that is quite shallow.
3. Coat each salmon fillet with the pistachio mixture after brushing it with Dijon mustard and then setting it aside.
4. Put the fillets on a baking sheet that has been lined with parchment paper.
5. Olive oil should be drizzled over the top of each fillet.
6. Put the salmon in the oven and bake for fifteen minutes, or until the salmon is fully cooked and the crust is golden brown.
7. Lemon wedges should be served on a separate plate, as this is the preferred practice.

Per serving: Calories: 280kcal; Fat: 18g; Carbs: 7g; Protein: 25g; Sugar: 1g

115. *Orange Glazed Grilled Swordfish*

Preparation time: 15 minutes
Cooking time: 10 minutes
Servings: 4

Ingredients:

- 4 swordfish steaks
- Zest and juice of 2 oranges
- 2 tbsps low-sodium soy sauce
- 1 tbsp honey or a sugar substitute
- 1 tsp grated ginger
- 2 pieces garlic, crushed
- Fresh parsley for garnish

Directions:

1. Bring the temp. of the grill up to a med-high level.
2. In a bowl, blend the orange zest, orange juice, soy sauce, honey (or a sugar substitute), grated ginger, and smashed garlic by whisking them together.
3. Put your swordfish steaks on the grill and cook them for 4 to 5 minutes on all sides, or until they are fully done.
4. During the final few minutes of grilling, brush the orange glaze over the swordfish and set it aside.
5. Before delivering the dish, garnish it with pieces of fresh parsley.

Per serving: Calories: 300kcal; Fat: 12g; Carbs: 10g; Protein: 30g; Sugar: 7g

116. *Lemon Dill Baked Trout*

Preparation time: 10 minutes
Cooking time: 15 minutes
Servings: 4
Ingredients:

- 4 trout fillets
- 2 tbsps olive oil
- Zest and juice of 1 lemon
- 1 tbsp fresh dill, cut into small bits
- 1 tsp garlic powder

- Salt and black pepper as needed
- Lemon wedges for presenting

Directions:

1. Warm up your oven to 400 deg.F.
2. Placing the trout fillets on a baking sheet that has been lined with parchment paper.
3. In the bowl you have, blend the following components: olive oil, lemon zest, lemon juice, fresh dill that has been cut into small bits, garlic powder, salt, and black pepper.
4. Apply a light coating of the lemon-dill mixture to each fillet of fish.
5. Bake the trout for 15 minutes, or until it is completely cooked through.
6. It is advised that lemon wedges be served on a separate plate after the main course.

Per serving: Calories: 200kcal; Fat: 10g; Carbs: 0g; Protein: 25g; Sugar: 0g

117. *Dijon Mustard Baked Cod*

Preparation time: 15 minutes
Cooking time: 15 minutes
Servings: 4
Ingredients:

- 4 cod fillets
- 2 tbsps Dijon mustard
- 1 tbsp olive oil
- 1 tbsp fresh dill, cut into small bits
- 1 tsp garlic powder
- Salt and black pepper as needed
- Lemon wedges for presenting

Directions:

1. Warm up your oven to 400 deg.F.

2. Organize the fish fillets in a circle on the baking sheet that has been prepared with parchment paper.
3. Blend in a bowl the following components: Dijon mustard, olive oil, fresh dill that has been cut into small bits, garlic powder, salt, and black pepper together.
4. Coat each cod fillet with the mustard combination made using Dijon mustard.
5. Bake the fish for 15 minutes, or until it is completely cooked through.
6. It is advised that lemon wedges be served on a separate plate after the main course.

Per serving: Calories: 200kcal; Fat: 8g; Carbs: 1g; Protein: 25g; Sugar: 0g

118. *Mediterranean Baked Salmon*

Preparation time: 15 minutes
Cooking time: 15 minutes
Servings: 4
Ingredients:

- 4 salmon fillets
- 2 tbsps olive oil
- 2 tsps dried oregano
- 1 tsp dried thyme
- 1 tsp garlic powder
- 1 lemon, cut
- 1/2 cup cherry tomatoes, divided
- 1/4 cup feta cheese, crumbled
- Fresh parsley for garnish

Directions:

1. Warm up your oven to 400 deg.F.

2. On a baking sheet that has been lined with parchment paper, arrange the salmon fillets in a single layer.

3. Blend garlic powder, dried oregano, dried thyme, and olive oil in a bowl. Mix the entire ingredients.

4. Coat each salmon fillet well with the olive oil mixture using a brush.

5. Establish the salmon on top of the lemon slices, cherry tomatoes, and crumbled feta cheese.

6. Bake the salmon for fifteen minutes, or until it is completely cooked through.

7. Before delivering the dish, garnish it with pieces of fresh parsley.

Per serving: Calories: 280kcal; Fat: 18g; Carbs: 5g; Protein: 25g; Sugar: 2g

119. *Sesame Ginger Glazed Tuna Steak*

Preparation time: 10 minutes
Cooking time: 5 minutes
Servings: 4
Ingredients:

- 4 tuna steaks
- 2 tbsps low-sodium soy sauce
- 1 tbsp sesame oil
- 1 tbsp rice vinegar
- 1 tsp grated ginger
- 2 pieces garlic, crushed
- 1 tbsp sesame seeds for garnish
- Sliced green onions for garnish

Directions:

1. First, get the grill up to a high temp.
2. Blend some grated ginger, some soy sauce, some sesame oil, some rice vinegar, and some crushed garlic in a basin and whisk them together.

3. Cook tuna steaks on the grill for 2 to 3 minutes on all sides for med-rare, or for further if you prefer a more done texture.

4. During the final minute of grilling, apply the sesame ginger glaze on the tuna by brushing it on.

5. Prior to presenting, garnish with green onions and sesame seeds that have been cut into small bits into chunks.

Per serving: Calories: 250kcal; Fat: 12g; Carbs: 2g; Protein: 30g; Sugar: 0g

120. *Walnut-Crusted Baked Trout*

Preparation time: 15 minutes
Cooking time: 15 minutes
Servings: 4
Ingredients:

- 4 trout fillets
- 1/2 cup walnuts, finely cut into small bits
- 1/4 cup whole wheat breadcrumbs
- 1 tsp dried thyme
- 1 tsp garlic powder
- 2 tbsps Dijon mustard
- 1 tbsp olive oil
- Lemon wedges for presenting

Directions:

1. Warm up your oven to 400 deg.F.
2. Blend cut into small bits walnuts, breadcrumbs, dried thyme, and garlic powder in a plate that is quite shallow.

3. Coat each trout fillet with the walnut mixture after brushing it with Dijon mustard and then coating it with oil.

4. Put the fillets on a baking sheet that has been lined with parchment paper.

5. Olive oil should be drizzled over the top of every fillet.

6. Put the trout in the oven and bake for 15 minutes, or until the crust is golden brown and the trout is fully cooked.

7. Lemon wedges should be served on a separate plate, as this is the preferred practice.

Per serving: Calories: 270kcal; Fat: 16g; Carbs: 7g; Protein: 25g; Sugar: 1g

POULTRY RECIPES

Per serving: Calories: 320kcal; Fat: 25g; Carbs: 1g; Protein: 22g; Sugar: 0g

121. Garlic Parmesan Baked Chicken Wings

Preparation time: 15 minutes
Cooking time: 45 minutes
Servings: 4
Ingredients:

- 2 lbs chicken wings, split at joints, tips discarded
- 1/4 cup grated Parmesan cheese
- 2 tbsps olive oil
- 2 tsps garlic powder
- 1 tsp dried oregano
- 1 tsp dried basil
- Salt and black pepper as needed
- Fresh parsley for garnish

Directions:

1. Warm up your oven to 400 deg.F.
2. In a bowl, blend grated Parmesan cheese, olive oil, garlic powder, dried oregano, dried basil, salt, and black pepper. Mix the entire ingredients.
3. After the chicken wings have been patted dry, they should be coated with the Parmesan mixture.
4. Using a baking sheet that has been lined with parchment paper, put the wings on the sheet.
5. Bake for 45 minutes, or until the wings have a golden brown color and a crisp texture.
6. Before delivering the dish, garnish it with pieces of fresh parsley.

122. Greek Lemon Chicken with Vegetables

Preparation time: 20 minutes
Cooking time: 40 minutes
Servings: 4
Ingredients:

- 4 bone-in, skin-on chicken thighs
- 1 lb baby potatoes, divided
- 1 cup cherry tomatoes
- 1 red onion, cut into wedges
- 2 tbsps olive oil
- Zest and juice of 1 lemon
- 2 tsps dried oregano
- 3 pieces garlic, crushed
- Salt and black pepper as needed
- Fresh parsley for garnish

Directions:

1. Warm up your oven to 400 deg.F.
2. In a bowl, blend the following components: olive oil, lemon zest, lemon juice, dried oregano, crushed garlic, salt, and black pepper.
3. Arrange an assortment of ingredients on your baking sheet, including chicken thighs, baby potatoes, cherry tomatoes, and red onion wedges.
4. Apply the mixture of olive oil and lemon juice to the chicken and veggies and brush it on together.
5. Bake the chicken for 40 minutes, or until it reaches a golden brown color and is evenly cooked throughout.
6. Before delivering the dish, garnish it with pieces of fresh parsley.

Per serving: Calories: 350kcal; Fat: 18g; Carbs: 25g; Protein: 22g; Sugar: 3g

123. Almond-Crusted Turkey Cutlets

Preparation time: 15 minutes
Cooking time: 20 minutes
Servings: 4
Ingredients:

- 4 turkey cutlets
- 1/2 cup almonds, finely cut into small bits
- 1/4 cup whole wheat breadcrumbs
- 1 tsp dried thyme
- 1 tsp garlic powder
- 2 tbsps Dijon mustard
- 1 tbsp olive oil
- Lemon wedges for presenting

Directions:

1. Warm up your oven to 400 deg.F.
2. Almonds that have been cut into small bits, breadcrumbs, dried thyme, and garlic powder should be mixed together in a shallow dish.
3. Prepare each turkey cutlet by brushing it with Dijon mustard and then coating it with the almond coating.
4. Using a baking sheet that has been prepared with parchment paper, put the cutlets on the sheet.
5. Olive oil should be drizzled over the top of every cutlet.
6. Put the turkey in the oven and bake for 20 minutes, or until the turkey is fully cooked and the crust is golden brown.

7. Lemon wedges should be served on a separate plate, as this is the preferred practice.

Per serving: Calories: 280kcal; Fat: 15g; Carbs: 7g; Protein: 25g; Sugar: 1g

124. Lemon Rosemary Grilled Chicken Thighs

Preparation time: 15 minutes
Cooking time: 20 minutes
Servings: 4
Ingredients:

- 4 bone-in, skinless chicken thighs
- Zest and juice of 1 lemon
- 2 tbsps olive oil
- 1 tbsp fresh rosemary, cut into small bits
- 2 pieces garlic, crushed
- Salt and black pepper as needed

Directions:

1. In a bowl, blend the following components: lemon zest, lemon juice, olive oil, fresh rosemary that has been cut into small bits, garlic that has been crushed, salt, and black pepper.
2. Put the chicken thighs in the plastic bag that can be sealed, and then pour the marinade over them. Next, put the bag in the fridge for close to half an hour.
3. Bring the temp. of the grill up to a med-high level.
4. Cook chicken thighs on the grill for 10 to 12 minutes on all sides, or until the internal temp. reaches 165 deg.F.
5. Please allow the chicken to rest for a couple of minutes before delivering it to the audience.

Per serving: Calories: 250kcal; Fat: 15g; Carbs: 1g; Protein: 26g; Sugar: 0g

125. Orange Ginger Glazed Chicken Stir-Fry

Preparation time: 20 minutes
Cooking time: 15 minutes
Servings: 4
Ingredients:

- 1 lb boneless, skinless chicken breast, that is finely cut
- 2 tbsps low-sodium soy sauce
- Zest and juice of 1 orange
- 1 tbsp honey or a sugar substitute
- 1 tbsp fresh ginger, grated
- 2 pieces garlic, crushed
- 1 tbsp cornstarch
- 2 tbsps vegetable oil
- 2 cups broccoli florets
- 1 red bell pepper, cut
- 1 cup snap peas
- Cooked brown rice for presenting

Directions:

1. To prepare the sauce, blend the following components in a bowl: soy sauce, orange zest, orange juice, honey (or a sugar replacement), grated ginger, smashed garlic, and cornstarch until everything is thoroughly combined.
2. To begin, bring the vegetable oil in your wok or big skillet to a high temp.
3. Include the chicken slices, then stir-fry them for 3 to 4 minutes, until they are browned and cooked all the way through.
4. Put the snap peas, broccoli, and red bell pepper into the wok and stir in the

garlic. Stir-fry the vegetables for an extra 4 to 5 minutes, or until they are crisp-tender.
5. Drizzle the cooked chicken and vegetables with the sauce. All of the ingredients should be properly heated, and then they should be tossed together until they are completely coated.
6. Serve atop brown rice that has been cooked.

Per serving: Calories: 300kcal; Fat: 10g; Carbs: 25g; Protein: 25g; Sugar: 10g

126. Teriyaki Chicken and Vegetable Stir-Fry

Preparation time: 15 minutes
Cooking time: 15 minutes
Servings: 4
Ingredients:

- 1 lb boneless, skinless chicken breast, that is finely cut
- 1 cup broccoli florets
- 1 bell pepper, cut
- 1 carrot, julienned
- 1 cup snap peas
- 2 tbsps low-sodium soy sauce
- 1 tbsp honey or a sugar substitute
- 1 tbsp rice vinegar
- 1 tsp sesame oil
- 1 tsp grated ginger
- 2 pieces garlic, crushed
- 2 tbsps vegetable oil
- Sesame seeds for garnish
- Green onions for garnish

Directions:

1. To make your sauce, blend the following components in a bowl: soy sauce, honey (or a sugar replacement), rice vinegar, sesame oil, grated ginger, and smashed garlic.

2. To begin, bring the vegetable oil in your wok or big skillet to a high temp.

3. Include the chicken slices, then stir-fry them for 3 to 4 minutes, until they are browned and cooked all the way through.

4. Include snap peas, broccoli, bell pepper, and carrots that have been julienned to the wok. Continue cooking. Stir-fry the vegetables for an extra 4 to 5 minutes, or until they are crisp-tender.

5. Drizzle the cooked chicken and vegetables with the sauce. To ensure that everything is evenly covered and heated thoroughly, toss everything together.

6. Sesame seeds and sliced green onions should be used as sprinkles for garnish.

7. Serve atop brown rice that has been cooked.

Per serving: Calories: 300kcal; Fat: 10g; Carbs: 25g; Protein: 25g; Sugar: 10g

127. Chicken and Vegetable Skewers

Preparation time: 20 minutes
Cooking time: 15 minutes
Servings: 4
Ingredients:

- 1 lb boneless, skinless chicken breast, that is cut into cubes
- 1 zucchini, cut
- 1 bell pepper, cut into chunks
- 1 red onion, cut into chunks
- 2 tbsps olive oil
- 1 tsp dried oregano
- 1 tsp garlic powder
- Salt and black pepper as needed
- Lemon wedges for presenting

Directions:

1. Bring the temp. of the grill up to a med-high level.

2. In a bowl, blend the following components: garlic powder, dried oregano, olive oil, and salt and black pepper until thoroughly blended.

3. Thread each of the following components onto skewers: chicken cubes, zucchini slices, bell pepper chunks, and red onion chunks.

4. Apply the olive oil mixture on the skewers and brush them.

5. Put the chicken on the grill and cook it for 10 to 12 minutes, turning it occasionally, until it is fully cooked and the vegetables are soft.

6. It is advised that lemon wedges be served on a separate plate after the main course.

Per serving: Calories: 220kcal; Fat: 10g; Carbs: 5g; Protein: 25g; Sugar: 2g

128. Turkey and Spinach Stuffed Peppers

Preparation time: 20 minutes
Cooking time: 25 minutes
Servings: 4
Ingredients:

- 4 big bell peppers, divided and seeds taken out

- 1 lb ground turkey
- 1 cup fresh spinach, cut into small bits
- 1 cup cherry tomatoes, cubed
- 1/2 cup onion, finely cut into small bits
- 2 pieces garlic, crushed
- 1 tsp dried oregano
- 1 tsp paprika
- Salt and black pepper as needed
- 1 cup low-sodium tomato sauce
- 1/2 cup feta cheese, crumbled

Directions:

1. Warm up your oven to 375 deg.F.
2. Cook the ground turkey in your skillet until it has a browned appearance. Take off any surplus fat.
3. In your skillet, include the following components: cut into small bits spinach, cubed cherry tomatoes, cut into small bits onion, smashed garlic, dried oregano, paprika, salt, and black pepper. Continue cooking for an extra 3 to 4 minutes until the vegetables have become more tender.
4. Put a portion of the turkey and veggie mixture inside of each half of the bell pepper.
5. Pour tomato sauce over the peppers that have been filled.
6. Put the peppers in the oven and bake for 25 minutes, or until they are soft.
7. Prior to presenting, sprinkle some crumbled feta cheese over the top of the cheese.

Per serving: Calories: 300kcal; Fat: 12g; Carbs: 20g; Protein: 25g; Sugar: 10g

129. Honey Mustard Glazed Chicken Drumsticks

Preparation time: 15 minutes
Cooking time: 40 minutes
Servings: 4
Ingredients:

- 8 chicken drumsticks
- 1/4 cup Dijon mustard
- 2 tbsps honey or a sugar substitute
- 1 tbsp olive oil
- 1 tsp garlic powder
- Salt and black pepper as needed
- Fresh parsley for garnish

Directions:

1. Warm up your oven to 400 deg.F.
2. In a bowl, blend the Dijon mustard, honey (or sugar alternative), olive oil, garlic powder, salt, and black pepper by continuously whisking the entire components together.
3. Coat the chicken drumsticks with the honey mustard mixture after patting them dry with paper towels.
4. Put the drumsticks on a baking sheet that has been lined with parchment paper.
5. Bake the chicken for 40 minutes, or until it reaches a golden brown color and is evenly cooked throughout.
6. Before delivering the dish, garnish it with pieces of fresh parsley.

Per serving: Calories: 280kcal; Fat: 15g; Carbs: 8g; Protein: 26g; Sugar: 7g

130. Baked Chicken Breast with Herbs

Preparation time: 10 minutes
Cooking time: 25 minutes
Servings: 4
Ingredients:

- 4 boneless, skinless chicken breasts
- 2 tbsps olive oil
- 1 tsp dried thyme
- 1 tsp dried rosemary
- 1 tsp garlic powder
- Salt and black pepper as needed
- Lemon wedges for presenting

Directions:

1. Warm up your oven to 400 deg.F.
2. On a baking sheet that has been lined with parchment paper, arrange the chicken breasts in a single layer.
3. In a bowl, blend the following components: garlic powder, salt, black pepper, dried thyme, and dried rosemary; olive oil; and garlic powder.
4. Coat each chicken breast with the herb mixture using a combination brush.
5. Put the chicken in the oven and bake for 25 minutes, or until the flesh is completely heated through and the middle is no longer pink.
6. It is advised that lemon wedges be served on a separate plate after the main course.

Per serving: Calories: 200kcal; Fat: 9g; Carbs: 0g; Protein: 28g; Sugar: 0g

131. Cilantro Lime Grilled Chicken

Preparation time: 15 minutes

Cooking time: 15 minutes
Servings: 4
Ingredients:

- 4 boneless, skinless chicken breasts
- 1/4 cup fresh cilantro, cut into small bits
- Zest and juice of 2 limes
- 2 tbsps olive oil
- 1 tsp cumin
- 1 tsp paprika
- Salt and black pepper as needed

Directions:

1. Blend cut into small bits cilantro, lime zest, lime juice, olive oil, cumin, paprika, salt, and black pepper in a bowl. Mix by hand until everything is evenly distributed.
2. The chicken breasts should be coated with a mixture of cilantro and lime.
3. Bring the temp. of the grill up to a med-high level.
4. Put your chicken breasts on the grill and cook them for 6 to 8 minutes on all sides, or until they are fully done.
5. Before delivering the chicken, the bird should be allowed to rest for a couple of minutes.

Per serving: Calories: 250kcal; Fat: 12g; Carbs: 1g; Protein: 30g; Sugar: 0g

132. Pesto Marinated Chicken Breast

Preparation time: 10 minutes
Cooking time: 15 minutes
Servings: 4
Ingredients:

- 4 boneless, skinless chicken breasts

- 1/2 cup basil pesto (store-bought or homemade)
- Zest and juice of 1 lemon
- 2 tbsps olive oil
- Salt and black pepper as needed

Directions:

1. Blend the following components in a bowl: olive oil, salt, basil pesto, lemon zest, lemon juice, and black pepper.
2. Apply the pesto mixture to the chicken breasts and coat them.
3. Bring the temp. of the grill up to a med-high level.
4. Put your chicken breasts on the grill and cook them for 6 to 8 minutes on all sides, or until they are fully done.
5. Before delivering the chicken, the bird should be allowed to rest for a couple of minutes.

Per serving: Calories: 300kcal; Fat: 18g; Carbs: 2g; Protein: 30g; Sugar: 0g

133. Cranberry Balsamic Glazed Chicken

Preparation time: 15 minutes
Cooking time: 30 minutes
Servings: 4
Ingredients:

- 4 bone-in, skin-on chicken thighs
- 1/2 cup cranberry sauce (sugar-free or low-sugar)
- 2 tbsps balsamic vinegar
- 1 tbsp olive oil
- 1 tsp dried rosemary
- Salt and black pepper as needed
- Fresh parsley for garnish

Directions:

1. Warm up your oven to 400 deg.F.
2. In a bowl, blend the cranberry sauce, balsamic vinegar, olive oil, dried rosemary, salt, and black pepper by whisking the entire components together.
3. Organize the chicken thighs one at a time on the baking sheet that has been prepared with parchment paper.
4. Apply the cranberry balsamic glaze to the chicken and thoroughly coat it.
5. Bake the chicken for 30 minutes or until it reaches a golden brown color and is evenly cooked throughout.
6. Before delivering the dish, garnish it with pieces of fresh parsley.

Per serving: Calories: 350kcal; Fat: 18g; Carbs: 20g; Protein: 22g; Sugar: 10g

134. Spinach and Feta Stuffed Chicken Breast

Preparation time: 20 minutes
Cooking time: 25 minutes
Servings: 4
Ingredients:

- 4 boneless, skinless chicken breasts
- 2 cups fresh spinach, cut into small bits
- 1/2 cup feta cheese, crumbled
- 1/4 cup sun-dried tomatoes, cut into small bits
- 2 pieces garlic, crushed
- 1 tsp dried oregano
- Salt and black pepper as needed
- 1 tbsp olive oil

Directions:

1. Warm up your oven to 400 deg.F.

2. In a bowl, blend the following components: cut into small bits spinach, crumbled feta cheese, sun-dried tomatoes, crushed garlic, dried oregano, salt, and black pepper.

3. Create a pocket in each of the chicken breasts.

4. Fill each chicken breast with a mixture of spinach and feta cheese.

5. Tie toothpicks around the pockets to secure them.

6. Coat the chicken breasts with olive oil using a scrub brush.

7. Bake the chicken for 25 minutes, or until the juices run clear and the chicken is fully done.

8. Before presenting, remove the toothpicks from the container.

Per serving: Calories: 300kcal; Fat: 15g; Carbs: 5g; Protein: 30g; Sugar: 2g

salt, and black pepper in the bowl. Continue mixing until everything is well distributed.

3. Organize the chicken thighs one at a time on the baking sheet that has been prepared with parchment paper.

4. Apply the paprika mixture to the chicken and rub it in.

5. Bake the chicken for 35 minutes, or until it reaches a golden brown color and is fully cooked.

6. Present instantly.

Per serving: Calories: 350kcal; Fat: 25g; Carbs: 1g; Protein: 26g; Sugar: 0g

135. Paprika Roasted Chicken Thighs

Preparation time: 10 minutes
Cooking time: 35 minutes
Servings: 4
Ingredients:

- 4 bone-in, skin-on chicken thighs
- 2 tsps paprika
- 1 tsp garlic powder
- 1 tsp onion powder
- 1 tsp dried thyme
- 1 tbsp olive oil
- Salt and black pepper as needed

Directions:

1. Warm up your oven to 400 deg.F.

2. Blend the paprika, garlic powder, onion powder, dried thyme, olive oil,

SOUP AND STEW RECIPES

136. Minestrone Soup with Quinoa

Preparation time: 15 minutes
Cooking time: 30 minutes
Servings: 6
Ingredients:

- 1 cup quinoa, washed
- 2 tbsps olive oil
- 1 onion, cut into small bits
- 2 carrots, cubed
- 2 celery stalks, cut into small bits
- 3 pieces garlic, crushed
- 1 tin (14 oz) cubed tomatoes
- 1 tin (15 oz) kidney beans, that is drained and washed
- 1 zucchini, cubed
- 1 tsp dried oregano
- 1 tsp dried basil
- 1/2 tsp dried thyme
- 6 cups vegetable broth
- Salt and black pepper as needed
- Fresh parsley for garnish

Directions:

1. Prepare the quinoa in your pot as per to the guidelines on the package. Put away.
2. Bring your olive oil to a temp. that is right in the middle in your big soup pot.
3. Include pieces of cut into small bits onion, cubed carrots, cut into small bits celery, and garlic that have been compressed. For vegetables to become more tender, sauté them.
4. Incorporate cut into small bits tomatoes, kidney beans, zucchini, dried oregano, dried basil, and dried thyme into the mixture. Give it a good stir.
5. After adding the vegetable broth, bring the soup to a boil and continue cooking.
6. Reduce the temp., cover, and let it simmer for 15 to 20 minutes.
7. Stir in the quinoa that has been cooked and flavor with salt and black pepper.
8. Continue to simmer for an extra 5 minutes.
9. Fresh parsley should be used as a garnish before presenting.

Per serving: Calories: 250kcal; Fat: 7g; Carbs: 40g; Protein: 10g; Sugar: 5g

137. Spinach and Chickpea Stew

Preparation time: 15 minutes
Cooking time: 25 minutes
Servings: 4
Ingredients:

- 1 tbsp olive oil
- 1 onion, cut into small bits
- 3 pieces garlic, crushed
- 1 tin (15 oz) chickpeas, that is drained and washed
- 1 tin (14 oz) cubed tomatoes
- 4 cups baby spinach
- 1 tsp ground cumin
- 1/2 tsp ground coriander
- 1/2 tsp smoked paprika
- Salt and black pepper as needed

- Lemon wedges for presenting

Directions:

1. Bring the olive oil to a temp. just in the middle of your big pot.
2. Include garlic that has been smashed by hand and sliced onion. To ensure that the onion is completely translucent, sauté it.
3. Chickpeas, cubed tomatoes, baby spinach, ground cumin, ground coriander, and smoked paprika should all be included in the cooking process. Give it a good stir.
4. Simmer for 15 to 20 minutes, or until the spinach has wilted and the flavors have been sufficiently combined.
5. Flavor with salt and black pepper.
6. It is advised that lemon wedges be served on a separate plate after the main course.

Per serving: Calories: 200kcal; Fat: 6g; Carbs: 30g; Protein: 8g; Sugar: 5g

138.   *Cabbage and Sausage Soup*

Preparation time: 20 minutes
Cooking time: 35 minutes
Servings: 6
Ingredients:

- 1 lb turkey sausage, cut
- 1 tbsp olive oil
- 1 onion, cut into small bits
- 3 pieces garlic, crushed
- 1 small head cabbage, shredded
- 3 carrots, cut
- 1 tin (14 oz) cubed tomatoes
- 6 cups chicken broth (low-sodium)

- 1 tsp dried thyme
- Salt and black pepper as needed
- Fresh parsley for garnish

Directions:

1. Bring the olive oil to a temp. just in the middle of your big pot.
2. Include the turkey sausage that has been cut, and make sure it is browned. When you have removed it from the pot, put it away.
3. Put the cut into small bits onion and garlic that has been crushed into the same pot. To ensure that the onion is completely translucent, sauté it.
4. Include grated cabbage, carrots that have been cut into small bits into pieces, cubed tomatoes, chicken stock, dried thyme, and sausage that has been cooked.
5. Bring the soup to a boil, then decrease the temp. and let it simmer for quarter to half an hour.
6. Flavor with salt and black pepper.
7. Before delivering the dish, garnish it with pieces of fresh parsley.

Per serving: Calories: 280kcal; Fat: 14g; Carbs: 20g; Protein: 18g; Sugar: 8g

139.   *Moroccan Spiced Lentil Soup*

Preparation time: 15 minutes
Cooking time: 30 minutes
Servings: 6
Ingredients:

- 1 cup dried red lentils, washed
- 2 tbsps olive oil
- 1 onion, cut into small bits
- 2 carrots, cubed
- 2 celery stalks, cut into small bits

- 3 pieces garlic, crushed
- 1 tsp ground cumin
- 1 tsp ground coriander
- 1/2 tsp ground turmeric
- 1/2 tsp cinnamon
- 1 tin (14 oz) cubed tomatoes
- 6 cups vegetable broth
- Salt and black pepper as needed
- Fresh cilantro for garnish
- Lemon wedges for presenting

Directions:

1. Prepare the red lentils in your pot as per to the guidelines on the package. Put away.
2. Bring your olive oil to a temp. that is right in the middle in your big soup pot.
3. Include pieces of cut into small bits onion, cubed carrots, cut into small bits celery, and garlic that have been compressed. For vegetables to become more tender, sauté them.
4. Include cinnamon, ground cumin, ground coriander, and ground turmeric to the mixture and stir to blend.
5. Include cubed tomatoes, red lentils that have been cooked, and vegetable broth in the recipe. Give it a good stir.
6. Afterwards, bring the soup to a simmer and allow it to cook for 20 to 25 minutes.
7. Include some salt and black pepper with the flavoring.
8. Prepare the dish by garnishing it with fresh cilantro and serving it with wedges of lemon.

Per serving: Calories: 240kcal; Fat: 7g; Carbs: 35g; Protein: 12g; Sugar: 5g

140. *Chicken and Vegetable Soup*

Preparation time: 15 minutes
Cooking time: 30 minutes
Servings: 6
Ingredients:

- 1 lb boneless, skinless chicken breasts, that is cooked and shredded
- 2 tbsps olive oil
- 1 onion, cut into small bits
- 2 carrots, cut
- 2 celery stalks, cut into small bits
- 3 pieces garlic, crushed
- 8 cups chicken broth (low-sodium)
- 1 cup green beans, that is cut into 1-inch pieces
- 1 cup corn kernels (fresh or frozen)
- 1 tsp dried thyme
- 1 tsp dried rosemary
- Salt and black pepper as needed
- Fresh parsley for garnish

Directions:

1. Bring the olive oil to a temp. just in the middle of your big pot.
2. Secondly, incorporate cut into small bits onion, cut into small bits carrots, cut into small bits celery, and smashed garlic into the mixture. For vegetables to become more tender, sauté them.
3. Afterwards, pour in your chicken broth and bring the mixture to a simmer.
4. A mixture of shredded chicken, green beans, corn, dried thyme, and dry rosemary should be introduced. Give it a good stir.
5. Flavor with salt and black pepper.

6. Simmer for 15 to 20 minutes, or until the vegetables grow soft.

7. Before delivering the dish, garnish it with pieces of fresh parsley.

Per serving: Calories: 220kcal; Fat: 8g; Carbs: 15g; Protein: 20g; Sugar: 5g

141. Tomato Basil Soup with Roasted Red Pepper

Preparation time: 15 minutes

Cooking time: 25 minutes

Servings: 4

Ingredients:

- 2 tbsps olive oil
- 1 onion, cut into small bits
- 3 pieces garlic, crushed
- 2 cans (14 oz each) cubed tomatoes
- 1 tin (12 oz) roasted red peppers, that is drained
- 4 cups vegetable broth
- 1 tsp dried basil
- Salt and black pepper as needed
- Fresh basil for garnish

Directions:

1. Bring the olive oil to a temp. just in the middle of your big pot.

2. Include garlic that has been crushed by hand and cut into small bits onion. To ensure that the onion is completely transparent, sauté it.

3. Include dried basil, cubed tomatoes, roasted red peppers, and vegetable broth to the aforementioned ingredients. Give it a good stir.

4. Bring the soup to a boil, then decrease the temp. and let it simmer for 15 minutes.

5. Blend the soup until it is completely smooth using a blender.

6. Flavor with salt and black pepper.

7. Before delivering the dish, garnish it with plenty of fresh basil.

Per serving: Calories: 180kcal; Fat: 9g; Carbs: 20g; Protein: 4g; Sugar: 8g

142. Butternut Squash and Carrot Soup

Preparation time: 15 minutes

Cooking time: 30 minutes

Servings: 4

Ingredients:

- 1 butternut squash, skinned, seeded, and cubed
- 4 carrots, skinned and cut into small bits
- 1 onion, cut into small bits
- 3 pieces garlic, crushed
- 1 tbsp olive oil
- 4 cups vegetable broth
- 1 tsp ground ginger
- 1/2 tsp ground cinnamon
- Salt and black pepper as needed
- Pumpkin seeds for garnish (optional)

Directions:

1. Bring the olive oil to a temp. just in the middle of your big pot.

2. Include garlic that has been smashed by hand and sliced onion. To ensure that the onion is completely translucent, sauté it.

3. Butternut squash that has been cubed, carrots that have been cut into small bits, vegetable broth, ground ginger,

and ground cinnamon should be included.

4. Bring to a boil, then decrease the temp. to a simmer and continue cooking for 20 to 25 minutes, or until the veggies are cooked.

5. Blend the soup until it is completely smooth using a blender.

6. Flavor with salt and black pepper.

7. If desired, garnish with pumpkin seeds of your choice.

Per serving: Calories: 180kcal; Fat: 4g; Carbs: 35g; Protein: 3g; Sugar: 8g

143. Chicken and Brown Rice Soup

Preparation time: 15 minutes
Cooking time: 40 minutes
Servings: 6
Ingredients:

- 1 lb boneless, skinless chicken breasts, that is cooked and shredded
- 1 tbsp olive oil
- 1 onion, cut into small bits
- 2 carrots, cut
- 2 celery stalks, cut into small bits
- 3 pieces garlic, crushed
- 1 cup brown rice, cooked
- 8 cups chicken broth (low-sodium)
- 1 tsp dried thyme
- Salt and black pepper as needed
- Fresh parsley for garnish

Directions:

1. Bring the olive oil to a temp. just in the middle of your big pot.

2. Secondly, incorporate cut into small bits onion, cut into small bits carrots,

cut into small bits celery, and smashed garlic into the mixture. For vegetables to become more tender, sauté them.

3. Afterwards, pour in your chicken broth and bring the mixture to a simmer.

4. Incorporate shredded chicken, brown rice that has been cooked, dried thyme, salt, and black pepper into the mixture. Give it a good stir.

5. Simmer for 25 to 30 minutes, or until the flavors have merged.

6. You may need to adjust the flavoring.

7. Before delivering the dish, garnish it with pieces of fresh parsley.

Per serving: Calories: 280kcal; Fat: 8g; Carbs: 25g; Protein: 25g; Sugar: 3g

144. Vegetable and Barley Soup

Preparation time: 20 minutes
Cooking time: 45 minutes
Servings: 6
Ingredients:

- 1 cup pearl barley, washed
- 2 tbsps olive oil
- 1 onion, cut into small bits
- 2 carrots, cubed
- 2 celery stalks, cut into small bits
- 3 pieces garlic, crushed
- 1 zucchini, cubed
- 1 tin (14 oz) cubed tomatoes
- 8 cups vegetable broth
- 1 tsp dried thyme
- Salt and black pepper as needed
- Fresh dill for garnish

Directions:

1. Start by cooking pearl barley in your pot as per to the guidelines on the package. Put away.
2. Bring your olive oil to a temp. that is right in the middle in your big soup pot.
3. Include pieces of cut into small bits onion, cubed carrots, cut into small bits celery, and garlic that have been compressed. For vegetables to become more tender, sauté them.
4. The fourth step is to incorporate cubed zucchini, salt, cubed tomatoes, pearl barley that has been boiled, vegetable broth, dried thyme, and black pepper. Give it a good stir.
5. After bringing the soup to a boil, decrease the temp. and let it simmer for half an hour.
6. You may need to adjust the flavoring.
7. Before presenting the dish, garnish it with plenty of fresh dill.

Per serving: Calories: 220kcal; Fat: 6g; Carbs: 40g; Protein: 6g; Sugar: 5g

145. Shrimp and Vegetable Gumbo

Preparation time: 20 minutes
Cooking time: 35 minutes
Servings: 4
Ingredients:

- 1 lb shrimp, skinned and deveined
- 2 tbsps olive oil
- 1 onion, cut into small bits
- 1 bell pepper, cubed
- 2 celery stalks, cut into small bits
- 3 pieces garlic, crushed

- 1 tin (14 oz) cubed tomatoes
- 4 cups chicken broth (low-sodium)
- 1 tbsp Cajun flavoring
- 1 tsp dried thyme
- Salt and black pepper as needed
- Green onions for garnish
- Cooked brown rice for presenting

Directions:

1. Bring the olive oil to a temp. just in the middle of your big pot.
2. Secondly, incorporate cut into small bits onion, cubed bell pepper, cut into small bits celery, and smashed garlic into the mixture. For vegetables to become more tender, sauté them.
3. The third step is to incorporate cubed tomatoes, chicken stock, Cajun flavoring, dried thyme, salt, and black pepper into the mixture. Give it a good stir.
4. Decrease the temp. to a simmer and allow the gumbo to cook for 20 to 25 minutes.
5. Include the shrimp, then continue cooking for an extra 5 to 7 minutes, or until the shrimp turned pink and are fully cooked.
6. You may need to adjust the flavoring.
7. Serve atop brown rice that has been cooked, and then garnish with green onions that have been cut into small bits.

Per serving: Calories: 300kcal; Fat: 10g; Carbs: 25g; Protein: 25g; Sugar: 5g

146. Broccoli and Cheddar Soup

Preparation time: 15 minutes
Cooking time: 25 minutes

Servings: 4
Ingredients:

- 4 cups broccoli florets
- 1 tbsp olive oil
- 1 onion, cut into small bits
- 2 carrots, cubed
- 3 pieces garlic, crushed
- 4 cups vegetable broth
- 1 cup sharp cheddar cheese, shredded
- 1 cup low-fat milk
- 2 tbsps whole wheat flour
- Salt and black pepper as needed
- Nutmeg for garnish (optional)

Directions:

1. Put broccoli in your pot and cook it until it is soft. Put away.
2. Bring your olive oil to a temp. that is right in the middle in your big soup pot.
3. Include cut into small bits onion, carrots that have been cubed, and garlic that has been smashed. For vegetables to become more tender, sauté them.
4. The fourth step is to sprinkle flour over the vegetables and then toss them together.
5. To prevent lumps from forming, gradually include the vegetable broth while mixing the mixture constantly.
6. Sixth, include broccoli that has been steamed to the pot.
7. In a separate bowl, blend shredded cheddar cheese and milk and stir until the mixture is smooth.
8. While constantly mixing, pour the cheese and milk combination into the soup you are previously making.

9. Simmer the soup for 10 to 15 minutes, or until it reaches the desired consistency.
10. Include some salt and black pepper to the finished dish.
11. If desired, garnish with a small amount of nutmeg on top.

Per serving: Calories: 280kcal; Fat: 15g; Carbs: 20g; Protein: 15g; Sugar: 8g

147. Turkey and White Bean Stew

Preparation time: 20 minutes
Cooking time: 35 minutes
Servings: 6
Ingredients:

- 1 lb ground turkey
- 1 tbsp olive oil
- 1 onion, cut into small bits
- 2 carrots, cubed
- 2 celery stalks, cut into small bits
- 3 pieces garlic, crushed
- 2 cans (15 oz each) white beans, that is drained and washed
- 1 tin (14 oz) cubed tomatoes
- 6 cups chicken broth (low-sodium)
- 1 tsp dried thyme
- 1 tsp dried rosemary
- Salt and black pepper as needed
- Fresh parsley for garnish

Directions:

1. Bring the olive oil to a temp. just in the middle of your big pot.
2. Include pieces of cut into small bits onion, cubed carrots, cut into small bits celery, and garlic that has been

compressed. For vegetables to become more tender, sauté them.

3. Include ground turkey, then continue to heat until it has a browned appearance.

4. Include the white beans, salt, cubed tomatoes, chicken broth, dried thyme, dried rosemary, and black pepper to the mixture and stir to blend.

5. Reduce the heat to a simmer and continue cooking the stew for an extra 25 to 30 minutes.

6. You may need to adjust the flavoring.

7. Before delivering the dish, garnish it with pieces of fresh parsley.

Per serving: Calories: 320kcal; Fat: 10g; Carbs: 30g; Protein: 25g; Sugar: 5g

148.   *Lemon Chicken Orzo Soup*

Preparation time: 15 minutes

Cooking time: 25 minutes

Servings: 4

Ingredients:

- 1 lb boneless, skinless chicken breasts, that is cooked and shredded
- 1 tbsp olive oil
- 1 onion, cut into small bits
- 2 carrots, cut
- 2 celery stalks, cut into small bits
- 3 pieces garlic, crushed
- 1 cup whole wheat orzo pasta
- 6 cups chicken broth (low-sodium)
- 1 lemon, juiced
- 1 tsp dried thyme
- Salt and black pepper as needed
- Fresh dill for garnish

Directions:

1. Bring the olive oil to a temp. just in the middle of your big pot.

2. Secondly, incorporate cut into small bits onion, cut into small bits carrots, cut into small bits celery, and smashed garlic into the mixture. For vegetables to become more tender, sauté them.

3. Afterwards, pour in your chicken broth and bring the mixture to a simmer.

4. Comprise the following components: shredded chicken, orzo pasta made with whole wheat, lemon juice, dried thyme, salt, and black pepper. Give it a good stir.

5. Simmer for 15 to 20 minutes, or until the orzo is done.

6. You may need to adjust the flavoring.

7. Before presenting the dish, garnish it with plenty of fresh dill.

Per serving: Calories: 300kcal; Fat: 8g; Carbs: 35g; Protein: 25g; Sugar: 3g

149.   *Black-Eyed Pea and Kale Stew*

Preparation time: 20 minutes

Cooking time: 40 minutes

Servings: 6

Ingredients:

- 2 cups dried black-eyed peas, soaked overnight
- 1 tbsp olive oil
- 1 onion, cut into small bits
- 3 pieces garlic, crushed
- 1 bell pepper, cubed
- 1 bunch kale, stems taken out & leaves cut into small bits

- 1 tin (14 oz) cubed tomatoes
- 6 cups vegetable broth
- 1 tsp smoked paprika
- 1 tsp cumin
- Salt and black pepper as needed
- Hot sauce for presenting (optional)

Directions:

1. Follow the instructions on the package to boil black-eyed peas that have been soaked in your pot. Put away.
2. Bring your olive oil to a temp. that is right in the middle in your big soup pot.
3. Include cut into small bits onion, garlic that has been smashed, and bell pepper that has been cubed. For vegetables to become more tender, sauté them.
4. Incorporate the cut into small bits greens, and then sauté it until it has wilted.
5. Include black-eyed peas that have been cooked, cubed tomatoes, vegetable broth, smoked paprika, cumin, salt, and black pepper, and stir after each addition.
6. Bring the stew to a simmer and allow it to cook for half an hour.
7. If necessary, adjust the flavoring. "
8. If necessary, serve with a small amount of your favorite hot sauce.

Per serving: Calories: 280kcal; Fat: 6g; Carbs: 45g; Protein: 15g; Sugar: 5g

150. Italian Wedding Soup with Turkey Meatballs

Preparation time: 25 minutes
Cooking time: 30 minutes
Servings: 6

Ingredients:
For Turkey Meatballs:

- 1 lb ground turkey
- 1/2 cup whole wheat breadcrumbs
- 1/4 cup grated Parmesan cheese
- 1 egg
- 1 tsp dried oregano
- 1 tsp dried basil
- Salt and black pepper as needed

For Soup:

- 1 tbsp olive oil
- 1 onion, cut into small bits
- 2 carrots, cut
- 2 celery stalks, cut into small bits
- 3 pieces garlic, crushed
- 8 cups chicken broth (low-sodium)
- 2 cups baby spinach
- 1 cup small pasta (such as orzo)
- Salt and black pepper as needed
- Fresh parsley for garnish

Directions:

1. Blend ground turkey, breadcrumbs, Parmesan cheese, an egg, dried oregano, dried basil, salt, and black pepper in a bowl. Repeat with the other ingredients. Create very little meatballs.
2. Bring the olive oil to a temp. just in the middle of your big pot.
3. Third, incorporate cut into small bits onion, cut into small bits carrots, cut into small bits celery, and smashed garlic into the mixture. For vegetables to become more tender, sauté them.
4. Include your chicken broth and bring the mixture to a boil after adding it.

5. The fifth step is to incorporate turkey meatballs, baby spinach, and little pasta. Give it a good stir.

6. The meatballs should be cooked and the pasta should be soft after a simmer for 15 to 20 minutes.

7. If necessary, adjust the flavoring.

8. Before delivering the dish, garnish it with pieces of fresh parsley.

Per serving: Calories: 280kcal; Fat: 12g; Carbs: 20g; Protein: 25g; Sugar: 3g

DESSERT RECIPES

151. Dark Chocolate-Dipped Strawberries

Preparation time: 15 minutes
Cooking time: 0 minutes
Servings: 4
Ingredients:

- 1 cup dark chocolate chips (that is 70% cocoa or higher)
- 1 pint strawberries, washed and dried

Directions:

1. Line a piece of parchment paper on a baking sheet.
2. Melt the dark chocolate in individual intervals of thirty seconds in the bowl that is appropriate for use in the microwave, mixing in between each interval.
3. While holding each strawberry by its stem, dip it into the chocolate that has been melted, making sure that approximately two-thirds of the strawberry is covered.
4. Organize the strawberries that have been dipped on the preparation tray.
5. Put the chocolate in the fridge for roughly half an hour, or until it has hardened, whichever comes first.

Per serving: Calories: 150kcal; Fat: 8g; Carbs: 20g; Protein: 2g; Sugar: 12g

152. Berry Parfait with Greek Yogurt

Preparation time: 10 minutes
Cooking time: 0 minutes
Servings: 2
Ingredients:

- 1 cup Greek yogurt (unsweetened)
- 1 cup mixed berries (strawberries, blueberries, raspberries)
- 1/4 cup cut into small bits almonds
- 1 tbsp honey (optional)

Directions:

1. You should begin by layering Greek yogurt, mixed berries, and cut into small bits almonds in the glass or bowl you are using.
2. Continue using the same method until the glass or bowl is completely full.
3. Before presenting, the honey should be drizzled on top, if necessary.

Per serving: Calories: 220kcal; Fat: 10g; Carbs: 20g; Protein: 15g; Sugar: 10g

153. Chia Seed Pudding with Berries

Preparation time: 5 minutes (plus overnight chilling)
Cooking time: 0 minutes
Servings: 2
Ingredients:

- 1/4 cup chia seeds
- 1 cup unsweetened almond milk
- 1 tbsp maple syrup or sugar-free sweetener
- 1/2 tsp vanilla extract
- Mixed berries for topping

Directions:

1. Put the chia seeds, almond milk, maple syrup (or another sugar-free

sweetener), and vanilla essence into a bowl and mix them together.

2. Give the mixture a thorough stir, making sure that the chia seeds are distributed evenly throughout the mixture.

3. Place a lid on the bowl and put it in the fridge for at least four hours or overnight.

4. Before presenting, give the chia pudding a good stir to ensure that it has a creamy consistency.

5. Before presenting the dish, garnish it with a mixture of berries.

Per serving: Calories: 150kcal; Fat: 8g; Carbs: 15g; Protein: 5g; Sugar: 3g

154. Lemon Poppy Seed Muffins with Almond Flour

Preparation time: 15 minutes
Cooking time: 20 minutes
Servings: 12
Ingredients:

- 2 cups almond flour
- 1/4 cup coconut flour
- 1/2 tsp baking soda
- 1/4 tsp salt
- Zest of 1 lemon
- 3 tbsps lemon juice
- 3 big eggs
- 1/4 cup melted coconut oil
- 1/3 cup sugar-free sweetener
- 1 tsp vanilla extract
- 1 tbsp poppy seeds

Directions:

1. After preheating the oven to 350 deg.F, prepare your muffin tin by lining it with paper liners.

2. The second step is to blend the almond flour, coconut flour, baking soda, and salt in a bowl and whisk them together.

3. The third step is to blend the lemon zest, lemon juice, eggs, melted coconut oil, sugar-free sweetener, and vanilla extract in a separate bowl. Blend thoroughly.

4. Include the liquid components to the dry components, and stir until the mixture is almost completely blended.

5. Gently incorporate the poppy seeds into the mixture.

6. Transfer the batter to your muffin tin, being sure to fill each cup approximately two-thirds of the way.

7. Bake for 20 minutes, or until a toothpick immersed into the center of the cake comes out cleaner than it was before.

8. Before delivering the muffins, allow them to cool down first.

Per serving: Calories: 160kcal; Fat: 14g; Carbs: 6g; Protein: 5g; Sugar: 1g

155. Avocado Chocolate Mousse

Preparation time: 10 minutes
Cooking time: 0 minutes
Servings: 4
Ingredients:

- 2 ripe avocados
- 1/4 cup unsweetened cocoa powder
- 1/4 cup almond milk
- 1/4 cup sugar-free sweetener
- 1 tsp vanilla extract

- Pinch of salt
- Fresh berries for topping

Directions:

1. Put the avocados, cocoa powder, almond milk, sugar-free sweetener, vanilla extract, and a bit of salt into a mixer and beat until everything is combined.
2. Whip until it is silky smooth and creamy.
3. Put the mousse in the fridge for close to 2 hours to chill.
4. Transfer the mixture to serving dishes, and before presenting it, you should garnish it with fresh berries.

Per serving: Calories: 180kcal; Fat: 15g; Carbs: 11g; Protein: 3g; Sugar: 1g

156. Sugar-Free Jello with Fresh Fruit

Preparation time: 5 minutes (plus chilling time)

Cooking time: 0 minutes

Servings: 4

Ingredients:

- 1 box sugar-free gelatin (flavor of your choice)
- 1 cup boiling water
- 1 cup cold water
- Mixed fresh fruit for topping

Directions:

1. To begin, dissolve the sugar-free gelatin in water that is boiling as per to the guidelines on the package.
2. Toss in ice water and stir.
3. Put the mixture in the fridge until the gelatin begins to thicken but has not yet completely set.
4. Gently include a concoction of fresh fruits.
5. Keep cooling until the mixture is completely set.
6. Serve when chilled.

Per serving: Calories: 10kcal; Fat: 0g; Carbs: 1g; Protein: 1g; Sugar: 0g

157. Baked Apples with Cinnamon and Walnuts

Preparation time: 10 minutes

Cooking time: 30 minutes

Servings: 4

Ingredients:

- 4 big apples, cored and divided
- 2 tbsps melted coconut oil
- 1 tsp ground cinnamon
- 1/4 cup cut into small bits walnuts
- 1 tbsp honey (optional)

Directions:

1. Warm up your oven to 350 deg.F.
2. Put the apple halves in the baking dish that you have prepared.
3. Blend ground cinnamon and melted coconut oil in the small bowl you have available.
4. Give the apples a little brushing with the mixture.
5. Finally, sprinkle some cut into small bits walnuts on top.
6. Cook for 25 to 30 minutes, or until the apples are soft.
7. Honey should be drizzled on top, if necessary, before presenting.

Per serving: Calories: 180kcal; Fat: 10g; Carbs: 25g; Protein: 1g; Sugar: 18g

158. Strawberry and Almond Butter Bites

Preparation time: 10 minutes
Cooking time: 0 minutes
Servings: 4
Ingredients:

- 1 cup fresh strawberries, hulled
- 1/4 cup almond butter
- 1 tbsp chia seeds

Directions:

1. Cut each strawberry in half lengthwise.
2. Disperse a small quantity of almond butter on one-half of each strawberry for each of the strawberries.
3. Sprinkle the almond butter with chia seeds and set aside.
4. Put the remaining half of the strawberry on top, thereby forming a sandwich that is suitable for nibbling.
5. Before presenting, chill the food in the fridge for a period of 30 minutes.

Per serving: Calories: 80kcal; Fat: 5g; Carbs: 7g; Protein: 2g; Sugar: 3g

159. Raspberry Coconut Chia Seed Pudding

Preparation time: 10 minutes (plus overnight chilling)
Cooking time: 0 minutes
Servings: 2
Ingredients:

- 1/4 cup chia seeds
- 1 cup unsweetened coconut milk
- 1/2 cup fresh raspberries
- 1 tbsp sugar-free sweetener
- Unsweetened shredded coconut for topping

Directions:

1. Blend chia seeds, coconut milk, fresh raspberries, and sugar-free sweetener in a bowl.
2. Give it a good stir, making sure that the chia seeds are dispersed evenly at all times.
3. Put a lid on the bowl and place it in the fridge for at least 4 hours or overnight.
4. Before presenting, give the chia pudding a good stir to ensure that it has a creamy consistency.
5. Before serving, sprinkle the dish with shredded coconut that has not been sweetened.

Per serving: Calories: 200kcal; Fat: 14g; Carbs: 14g; Protein: 5g; Sugar: 2g

160. Mango Sorbet with Lime Zest

Preparation time: 10 minutes
Cooking time: 0 minutes
Servings: 4
Ingredients:

- 2 cups frozen mango chunks
- 1/4 cup water
- 2 tbsps lime juice
- Zest of one lime

Directions:

1. Using a mixer, blend frozen mango chunks, water, and lime juice until the mixture is completely smooth.

2. The second step is to pour the mixture into the shallow dish you have and smooth it out evenly.

3. Put the mixture into the freezer for around 4 hours, mixing it with a fork every half an hour to break up the ice crystals.

4. After the ice has completely frozen, scoop it out and serve it, garnishing it with lime zest.

Per serving: Calories: 90kcal; Fat: 0g; Carbs: 23g; Protein: 1g; Sugar: 19g

161. Greek Yogurt with Honey and Nuts

Preparation time: 5 minutes
Cooking time: 0 minutes
Servings: 2
Ingredients:

- 1 cup Greek yogurt (unsweetened)
- 2 tbsps honey
- 2 tbsps cut into small bits mixed nuts (almonds, walnuts, or pistachios)

Directions:

1. Put a spoonful of Greek yogurt in your bowl.

2. Honey should be drizzled over the yogurt two.

3. Include some cut into small bits nuts to the top of the dish.

4. Perform a light mixing just before presenting.

Per serving: Calories: 200kcal; Fat: 10g; Carbs: 18g; Protein: 12g; Sugar: 15g

162. Coconut and Almond Energy Bites

Preparation time: 15 minutes
Cooking time: 0 minutes
Servings: 12
Ingredients:

- 1 cup rolled oats
- 1/2 cup unsweetened shredded coconut
- 1/2 cup almond butter
- 1/4 cup honey
- 1/4 cup cut into small bits almonds
- 1 tsp vanilla extract
- Pinch of salt

Directions:

1. Put the rolled oats, shredded coconut, almond butter, honey, sliced almonds, vanilla essence, and a bit of salt into a bowl and mix them together.

2. Mix till everything is completely blended.

3. Put the mixture in the fridge for a period of thirty minutes.

4. After the mixture has been refrigerated, roll it into bite-sized servings of energy.

5. Put the energy bites on a tray that has been lined with parchment paper, and then put the tray in the fridge for an extra half an hour before presenting them.

Per serving: Calories: 150kcal; Fat: 9g; Carbs: 15g; Protein: 4g; Sugar: 7g

163. Almond Flour Blueberry Muffins

Preparation time: 15 minutes
Cooking time: 25 minutes
Servings: 12
Ingredients:

- 2 cups almond flour
- 1/4 cup coconut flour
- 1/2 tsp baking soda
- 1/4 tsp salt
- 3 big eggs
- 1/4 cup coconut oil, melted
- 1/4 cup unsweetened almond milk
- 1/3 cup sugar-free sweetener
- 1 tsp vanilla extract
- 1 cup fresh or frozen blueberries

Directions:

1. After preheating the oven to 350 deg.F, prepare your muffin tin by lining it with paper liners.
2. Blend the almond flour, coconut flour, baking soda, and salt in a bowl and whisk them together.
3. Beat the eggs in a separate bowl and then include the melted coconut oil, almond milk, sugar-free sweetener, and vanilla extract. Blend thoroughly.
4. After adding the wet components to the dry components, stir the mixture until it is almost completely incorporated.
5. Include the blueberries and fold them in carefully.
6. Transfer the batter to your muffin tin, being sure to fill each cup approximately two-thirds of the way.
7. Put the dish in the oven and bake for around 25 minutes, or until a toothpick immersed into the center appears clean.
8. Before delivering the muffins, allow them to cool down first.

Per serving: Calories: 150kcal; Fat: 12g; Carbs: 7g; Protein: 5g; Sugar: 2g

164. Chocolate Avocado Pudding

Preparation time: 10 minutes
Cooking time: 0 minutes
Servings: 4
Ingredients:

- 2 ripe avocados
- 1/4 cup unsweetened cocoa powder
- 1/4 cup almond milk
- 1/4 cup sugar-free sweetener
- 1 tsp vanilla extract
- Pinch of salt
- Dark chocolate shavings for topping

Directions:

1. Put the avocados, cocoa powder, almond milk, sugar-free sweetener, vanilla extract, and a bit of salt into a mixer and beat until everything is combined.
2. Whip until it is silky smooth and creamy.
3. The pudding should be chilled in the fridge for close to an hour.
4. Transfer the mixture to serving dishes and sprinkle it with dark chocolate shavings before giving it to the audience.

Per serving: Calories: 180kcal; Fat: 15g; Carbs: 11g; Protein: 3g; Sugar: 1g

165. Mixed Berry Sorbet

Preparation time: 10 minutes (plus freezing time)

Cooking time: 0 minutes

Servings: 4

Ingredients:

- 3 cups mixed berries (strawberries, blueberries, raspberries)
- 1/4 cup water
- 2 tbsps lemon juice
- 1-2 tbsps sugar-free sweetener (adjust as needed)

Directions:

1. First, put the mixed berries, water, lemon juice, and sugar-free sweetener into a mixer and mix them together.
2. Blend until it is completely smooth.
3. Transfer the mixture to a plate that is shallow and spread it out in an even manner.
4. Put in the freezer for a total of 2 to 3 hours, whisking the mixture with a fork every half an hour to break up the ice crystals.
5. When it is completely frozen, scoop it out and then offer it.

Per serving: Calories: 40kcal; Fat: 0g; Carbs: 10g; Protein: 1g; Sugar: 5g

BEVERAGE RECIPES

166. Carrot and Orange Juice Blend

Preparation time: 5 minutes
Cooking time: 0 minutes
Servings: 2
Ingredients:

- 4 medium carrots, skinned and cut into small bits
- 2 oranges, skinned and segmented
- 1/2 inch ginger, skinned
- 1 cup water
- Ice cubes (optional)

Directions:

1. Put the cubed carrots, orange segments, ginger, and water in a mixer and blend until combined.
2. Blend until it is completely smooth.
3. Include ice cubes, if necessary, and then blend once more until the ingredients are completely blended.
4. Pour the mixture into glasses and relish it.

Per serving: Calories: 70kcal; Fat: 0g; Carbs: 17g; Protein: 1g; Sugar: 10g

167. Kale and Pineapple Smoothie

Preparation time: 5 minutes
Cooking time: 0 minutes
Servings: 2
Ingredients:

- 2 cups kale leaves, stems taken out
- 1 cup pineapple chunks (fresh or frozen)
- 1 banana
- 1/2 cup coconut water
- Ice cubes (optional)

Directions:

1. To begin, put the kale leaves, pineapple chunks, banana, and coconut water in a mixer and mix until combined.
2. Blend until it is completely smooth.
3. Include ice cubes, if necessary, and then blend once more until the ingredients are completely blended.
4. Pour the mixture into glasses and relish it.

Per serving: Calories: 130kcal; Fat: 1g; Carbs: 32g; Protein: 3g; Sugar: 18g

168. Spinach and Berry Protein Smoothie

Preparation time: 5 minutes
Cooking time: 0 minutes
Servings: 2
Ingredients:

- 2 cups fresh spinach leaves
- 1 cup mixed berries (strawberries, blueberries, raspberries)
- 1/2 cup Greek yogurt (unsweetened)
- 1 scoop vanilla protein powder
- 1 cup water or unsweetened almond milk
- Ice cubes (optional)

Directions:

1. Put the fresh spinach, mixed berries, Greek yogurt, vanilla protein powder, and water (or almond milk) into a

mixer and mix until everything is combined.

2. Blend until it is completely smooth.

3. Include ice cubes, if necessary, and then blend once more until the ingredients are completely blended.

4. Pour the mixture into glasses and enjoy it.

Per serving: Calories: 150kcal; Fat: 3g; Carbs: 18g; Protein: 15g; Sugar: 9g

169. *Watermelon and Lime Juice*

Preparation time: 5 minutes
Cooking time: 0 minutes
Servings: 2
Ingredients:

- 2 cups cubed watermelon
- Juice of 2 limes
- 1 cup cold water
- Ice cubes (optional)
- Fresh mint leaves for garnish

Directions:

1. Put the watermelon cubes, lime juice, and cold water into a mixer and mix them together well.

2. In a blender, blend until smooth.

3. If necessary, incorporate ice cubes, and then blend once more until the ingredients are completely blended.

4. Pour into glasses, garnish with fresh mint leaves, and serve with delight; serve immediately.

Per serving: Calories: 50kcal; Fat: 0g; Carbs: 13g; Protein: 1g; Sugar: 9g

170. *Apple Cider Vinegar Detox Drink*

Preparation time: 5 minutes
Cooking time: 0 minutes
Servings: 1
Ingredients:

- 1 tbsp apple cider vinegar
- 1 tbsp lemon juice
- 1 tsp honey (optional)
- 1 cup water
- Ice cubes (optional)

Directions:

1. Apple cider vinegar, lemon juice, honey (if using), and water should be combined in a glass and stirred together.

2. Mix until everything is completely blended.

3. If necessary, include ice cubes, and then give the mixture another toss before sipping.

Per serving: Calories: 10kcal; Fat: 0g; Carbs: 3g; Protein: 0g; Sugar: 2g

171. *Avocado and Kale Smoothie*

Preparation time: 5 minutes
Cooking time: 0 minutes
Servings: 2
Ingredients:

- 1 ripe avocado, skinned and pitted
- 1 cup kale leaves, stems taken out
- 1 banana
- 1/2 cup plain Greek yogurt (unsweetened)
- 1 cup water or unsweetened almond milk

- Ice cubes (optional)

Directions:

1. Put the ripe avocado, the kale leaves, the banana, the Greek yogurt, and the water (or almond milk) into a mixer and mix them together.
2. Blend until it is completely smooth.
3. Include ice cubes, if necessary, and then blend once more until the ingredients are completely blended.
4. Pour the mixture into glasses and enjoy it.

Per serving: Calories: 220kcal; Fat: 12g; Carbs: 25g; Protein: 7g; Sugar: 11g

172. Tropical Mango and Coconut Smoothie

Preparation time: 5 minutes
Cooking time: 0 minutes
Servings: 2
Ingredients:

- 1 cup frozen mango chunks
- 1/2 cup coconut milk (unsweetened)
- 1/2 cup plain Greek yogurt (unsweetened)
- 1 tbsp shredded coconut
- 1/2 tsp vanilla extract
- Ice cubes (optional)

Directions:

1. Put frozen mango chunks, shredded coconut, coconut milk, Greek yogurt, and vanilla essence in a mixer and mix until everything is combined.
2. Blend until it is completely smooth.
3. Include ice cubes, if necessary, and then blend once more until the ingredients are completely blended.

4. Pour the mixture into glasses and relish it.

Per serving: Calories: 180kcal; Fat: 10g; Carbs: 20g; Protein: 6g; Sugar: 14g

173. Blueberry and Almond Milk Smoothie

Preparation time: 5 minutes
Cooking time: 0 minutes
Servings: 2
Ingredients:

- 1 cup blueberries (fresh or frozen)
- 1 banana
- 1 cup unsweetened almond milk
- 1/4 cup rolled oats
- 1 tbsp almond butter
- Ice cubes (optional)

Directions:

1. Put the blueberries, banana, almond milk, rolled oats, and almond butter into a mixer and mix until everything is combined.
2. Blend until it is completely smooth.
3. Include ice cubes, if necessary, and then blend once more until the ingredients are completely blended.
4. Pour the mixture into glasses and enjoy it.

Per serving: Calories: 200kcal; Fat: 8g; Carbs: 30g; Protein: 5g; Sugar: 14g

174. Green Goddess Smoothie with Spinach and Pineapple

Preparation time: 5 minutes
Cooking time: 0 minutes
Servings: 2

Ingredients:

- 2 cups fresh spinach leaves
- 1 cup pineapple chunks (fresh or frozen)
- 1/2 cucumber, skinned and cut
- 1/2 avocado
- 1 cup unsweetened almond milk
- Ice cubes (optional)

Directions:

1. Put the fresh spinach, pineapple pieces, cucumber, avocado, and almond milk into a mixer and mix until everything is combined.
2. Blend until it is completely smooth.
3. Include ice cubes, if necessary, and then blend once more until the ingredients are completely blended.
4. Pour the mixture into glasses and relish it.

Per serving: Calories: 120kcal; Fat: 7g; Carbs: 15g; Protein: 3g; Sugar: 7g

175. Berry Blast Smoothie with Greek Yogurt

Preparation time: 5 minutes
Cooking time: 0 minutes
Servings: 2
Ingredients:

- 1 cup mixed berries (strawberries, blueberries, raspberries)
- 1 tbsp chia seeds
- 1/2 cup Greek yogurt (unsweetened)
- 1/2 cup water or your unsweetened almond milk
- Ice cubes (optional)

Directions:

1. Put a mixture of mixed berries, Greek yogurt, water (or almond milk), and chia seeds in a mixer and mix until combined.
2. Blend until it is completely smooth.
3. Include ice cubes, if necessary, and then blend once more until the ingredients are completely blended.
4. Pour the mixture into glasses and relish it.

Per serving: Calories: 120kcal; Fat: 5g; Carbs: 15g; Protein: 6g; Sugar: 7g

176. Cucumber and Mint Infused Water

Preparation time: 5 minutes (plus chilling time)
Cooking time: 0 minutes
Servings: 4
Ingredients:

- 1 cucumber, finely cut
- Handful of fresh mint leaves
- 4 cups water
- Ice cubes (optional)

Directions:

1. Put the cucumber slices and the fresh mint leaves in a pitcher and mix them together.
2. Include the water, and then stir it out.
3. Put the mixture in the fridge for close to 2 hours to allow the flavors to develop.
4. If necessary, serve the drink over ice cubes.

Per serving: Calories: 0kcal; Fat: 0g; Carbs: 0g; Protein: 0g; Sugar: 0g

177. Peach and Raspberry Smoothie

Preparation time: 5 minutes
Cooking time: 0 minutes
Servings: 2
Ingredients:

- 1 cup frozen peaches
- 1/2 cup raspberries
- 1/2 cup plain Greek yogurt (unsweetened)
- 1/2 cup water or your unsweetened almond milk
- 1 tbsp chia seeds
- Ice cubes (optional)

Directions:

1. Put the frozen peaches, raspberries, Greek yogurt, water (or almond milk), and chia seeds into a mixer and mix them together.
2. Blend until it is completely smooth.
3. Include ice cubes, if necessary, and then blend once more until the ingredients are completely blended.
4. Pour the mixture into glasses and enjoy it.

Per serving: Calories: 120kcal; Fat: 3g; Carbs: 18g; Protein: 6g; Sugar: 11g

178. Celery and Cucumber Green Juice

Preparation time: 5 minutes
Cooking time: 0 minutes
Servings: 2
Ingredients:

- 4 celery stalks
- 1 cucumber
- 1 green apple, cored
- 1 lemon, skinned
- 1/2 inch ginger, skinned
- Ice cubes (optional)

Directions:

1. Put the celery, cucumber, green apple, lemon, and ginger into a juicer and begin processing them.
2. Give the juice a strong stir.
3. If necessary, put ice cubes before presenting.

Per serving: Calories: 60kcal; Fat: 0g; Carbs: 15g; Protein: 1g; Sugar: 8g

179. Kiwi and Banana Smoothie

Preparation time: 5 minutes
Cooking time: 0 minutes
Servings: 2
Ingredients:

- 2 kiwis, skinned and cut
- 1 banana
- 1/2 cup plain Greek yogurt (unsweetened)
- 1/2 cup water or your unsweetened almond milk
- 1 tbsp honey (optional)
- Ice cubes (optional)

Directions:

1. First, put the kiwi slices, banana, Greek yogurt, water (or almond milk), and honey (if you're using it) into a mixer and mix them together.
2. Blend until it is completely smooth.
3. Include ice cubes, if necessary, and then blend once more until the ingredients are completely blended.

4. Pour the mixture into glasses and enjoy it.

Per serving: Calories: 130kcal; Fat: 1g; Carbs: 29g; Protein: 3g; Sugar: 17g

180. Orange and Ginger Turmeric Tea

Preparation time: 5 minutes
Cooking time: 0 minutes
Servings: 2
Ingredients:

- 2 cups hot water
- 2 orange slices
- 1 tsp grated ginger
- 1/2 tsp ground turmeric
- 1 tsp honey (optional)

Directions:

1. In a teapot, blend the orange slices, grated ginger, ground turmeric, and honey (if you are using it). Pour hot water over the mixture.
2. Steep for 3 to 5 minutes.
3. Strain the tea into mugs, and then savor the calming beverage.

Per serving: Calories: 10kcal; Fat: 0g; Carbs: 3g; Protein: 0g; Sugar: 1g

BALANCED LIFESTYLE

Maintaining a healthy lifestyle is not merely a desirable objective; rather, it is an absolute must, particularly when dealing with diabetes after the age of 50. This critical juncture in one's life calls for a comprehensive strategy that incorporates making judicious decisions regarding one's food, engaging in regular physical activity, practicing stress management, showing compassion to oneself, and maintaining an ongoing dedication to prevention. Through the smooth incorporation of these components into your daily routine, you will not only be able to keep up with a healthy diet for diabetics, but you will also be able to improve your entire well-being.

Physical Exercise

In the fight against diabetes, moving your body is like having a secret weapon. Keeping your sugar levels under control is not the only benefit of this practice; it is also like giving your heart and body a jolt of superhuman power! It is possible to make a significant effect by engaging in activities such as brisk walking, biking, swimming, or other simple exercises for nearly 150 minutes every week.

However, here is the catch: before beginning any kind of workout program, it is of the utmost importance to consult with your physician as soon as possible, particularly if you have any health problems.

Moving on, let's speak about how you might incorporate physical activity into your daily routine. Modifying even a few aspects of your daily routine can have a significant impact. If you want to get a little bit of exercise, try using the stairs instead of the elevator. Place your vehicle a little further away so that you can take pleasure in a short walk. Doing duties around the house that need you to move around counts as exercise.

Find things to do that cause you to feel pleased. Put on some music and get ready to dance if you are someone who enjoys dancing. It's possible that a stroll through the park is what you're looking for if you enjoy being outside. The most important thing is to keep going and to make it entertaining. The experience is similar to that of making a new acquaintance; you look forward to spending time with them, and it eventually becomes a routine part of your life. You should get a friend or join a local group if you are interested in doing it. When you exercise together, you can have more fun, and you can encourage and support one another.

Always keep in mind that relocation does not have to be a massive and complicated plan. In terms of your health, even the smallest of efforts can lead to significant improvements. Put on those sneakers that are comfortable, choose an activity that you enjoy doing, and get ready to have a good time while reaping the wellness advantages!

Stress Management

It is of utmost significance for those over the age of 50 who are adhering to a diabetic diet to take care of their stress. The amount of sugar that is present in your blood and how you feel in general might be influenced by stress. Take a look at some simple suggestions that will assist you in managing stress and maintaining your health:

1. **Deep Breaths:** In order to calm down, it is recommended that you take slow and deep breaths. Inhale through your nose, then breathe out through your mouth so that you can breathe. Try to do this task for a few minutes. Stress is alleviated, and you have a greater sense of relaxation as a result.

2. **Moving Around:** It is important to engage in activities that you enjoy and that require you to move your body, such as gardening, walking, or riding a bike. This particular form of physical activity makes you feel better. Attempt to complete it for around 150 minutes each and every week.

3. **Mindful Moments:** Spend some time paying attention to what is occurring in the present moment. You can accomplish this by concentrating on your breath or by listening to someone else guide you through the process. Having this makes you feel more relaxed and less stressed out.

4. **Good Sleep:** You should make sure that you obtain enough amount of quality sleep. Keeping your sleeping space comfortable and establishing a pattern before going to bed can be helpful. Sleep deprivation can make stress worse and can also have an effect on your blood sugars.

5. **Organize Your Time:** Make a plan for your day that is tailored to your needs and organize your time accordingly. The most difficult activities should be broken down into smaller portions and completed one at a time. It is acceptable to decline additional requests if you are experiencing feelings of being overly busy. If you are able to, offer assistance with the chores.

6. **Family and Friends Time:** Spend time with the people who are important to you, including your family and your friends. When you talk about how you're feeling with them, it can help you feel better. You are better able to deal with stress when you have supporting friends and family members.

7. **Fun and Hobbies:** Do something that you enjoy doing, such as reading, listening to music, or engaging in a pastime. This is the seventh and final point. It is possible to alleviate stress and feel better by engaging in activities that are enjoyable.

8. **Eat Healthy:** Eating a balanced diet that includes a wide variety of foods, such as fruits, vegetables, lean meats, whole grains, and healthy fats, is the eighth step in maintaining a healthy diet. Your body will benefit from this type of eating, and it may also make it simpler for you to deal with stress.

9. **Watch Stimulants:** Coffee and cigarettes are two examples of stimulants that should be avoided because they lead to increased anxiety. Selecting herbal teas or beverages that do not include caffeine can be beneficial in reducing levels of stress.

10. **Get Help if Needed:** If you feel that the stress you are experiencing is too much for you to handle, you might think about hiring a professional. Helpful methods of coping with stress that are tailored to your needs can be provided to you by a therapist or counselor.

11. **Laugh and Have Fun:** Make sure you give yourself time to engage in activities that bring you joy and laughter. It is possible to find relief from stress by doing things like watching a funny movie or spending time with individuals who are able to make you laugh.

12. **Let Go of Things You Can't Control:** Recognize that not everything can be flawless and let go of things that you are unable to control completely. When you are in need of assistance, it is OK to ask for it. Instead of focusing on things that you can alter, you should let go of things that are bringing you unnecessary tension.

Empathic Approach

Adopting a compassionate attitude toward oneself is necessary in order to successfully navigate the hurdles of treating diabetes after the age of 50. When one considers that alterations to one's lifestyle are an essential component of diabetes care and that there is a possibility of experiencing setbacks, patience and self-awareness become crucial partners. Recognizing and honoring even the most insignificant achievements can serve as a potent incentive to continue making excellent decisions.

Individuals are given the ability to play an active role in their own health by receiving education about diabetes management strategies and via maintaining awareness of the various treatment options available. A platform that allows for the sharing of experiences, the seeking of guidance, and the provision of mutual support is provided by connecting with others who are experiencing similar issues through support groups or online communities. This kind of connection is a vital resource on the trip.

Importance of Prevention

The management of diabetes after the age of 50 places a significant emphasis on prevention. Committing to a healthy lifestyle and making intelligent decisions regarding the foods that you eat can be extremely helpful in preventing or delaying issues that are connected with diabetes. Give top priority to consuming a diet that is well-balanced and includes a wide variety of fruits, vegetables, lean meats, whole grains, and healthy fats. When taking preventative measures, it is important to limit the consumption of sugary drinks, processed foods, and foods that are high in saturated and trans fats.

Regular monitoring of blood sugar levels, in conjunction with the assistance of healthcare practitioners, is beneficial in the process of building individualized programs for the management of diabetes. It is possible to maintain a high level of control over diabetes by taking prescription medications as directed and going in for regular checkups. This will help reduce the risk of developing problems.

CONCLUSION

To summarize, maintaining control of diabetes after the age of 50 calls for an approach that is both comprehensive and individualised, taking into account a wide range of aspects of life. A comprehensive examination of the complexities of type 2 diabetes, including its risk factors, the critical role that diet plays, and the relevance of tailored meal plans, has been presented in this book. In order to achieve a balanced lifestyle for those over the age of 50 who are coping with diabetes, we discussed the significance of both physical activity and stress management, as well as the value of taking an empathic attitude.

Future Perspectives

When you start your path of treating diabetes after the age of 50, it is important to keep in mind that this is a commitment to your health that will last a lifetime. You should keep incorporating the information that you have learned from this book into your everyday life. Recognize and appreciate the great improvements you've made, rejoice in each and every achievement, and accept that failures are a natural and inevitable part of the process. Maintain a level of awareness regarding the latest developments in diabetes management, establish connections with communities that offer support, and never undervalue the significance of leading a healthy lifestyle.

Progress in medical research may, in the not too distant future, result in the development of novel approaches and therapies for diabetes. A proactive approach to remaining updated about these advancements should be taken, and you should work along with your healthcare team to incorporate any changes that could be useful into your management plan.

When it comes down to it, the way diabetes is managed after the age of 50 is different for each and every person. Not only will your dedication to leading a healthy lifestyle, regularly checking your condition, and taking preventative measures aid to the management of your diabetes, but it will also contribute to your general health and well-being. I hope that your journey is filled with resiliency, empowerment, and a quality of life that is blossoming like never before.

APPENDIX

30 Days Meal Plan

Day	Breakfast	Lunch	Dinner	Dessert
1	Quinoa Breakfast Porridge with Almonds	Whole Wheat Pasta with Tomato & Basil Sauce	Bulgur Pilaf with Mixed Vegetables	Baked Apples with Cinnamon and Walnuts
2	Sweet Potato Hash with Poached Eggs	Teriyaki Glazed Tilapia	Coconut Lime Shrimp Stir-Fry	Dark Chocolate-Dipped Strawberries
3	Vegetable Omelet with Spinach and Tomatoes	Herbed Grilled Pork Chops	Stuffed Bell Peppers with Lean Ground Beef	Berry Parfait with Greek Yogurt
4	Almond Butter & Banana Sandwich	Garlic Butter Shrimp and Broccoli	Spinach and Ricotta Stuffed Bell Peppers	Coconut and Almond Energy Bites
5	Berry Smoothie Bowl with Chia Seeds	Mediterranean Baked Salmon	Lemon Rosemary Grilled Chicken Thighs	Chia Seed Pudding with Berries
6	Spinach and Feta Frittata	Beef and Vegetable Stir-Fry	Coconut Lime Shrimp Stir-Fry	Sugar-Free Jello with Fresh Fruit
7	Cucumber and Tomato Breakfast Salad	Mushroom and Spinach Stuffed Pork Tenderloin	Orange Glazed Grilled Swordfish	Mixed Berry Sorbet
8	Cottage Cheese Pancakes with Berries	Lemon Dill Baked Trout	Garlic Parmesan Baked Chicken Wings	Almond Flour Blueberry Muffins
9	Broccoli and Cheese Egg Muffins	Teriyaki Glazed Tilapia	Greek Salad with Grilled Lamb	Avocado Chocolate Mousse
10	Avocado and Egg Breakfast Bowl	Herb-Roasted Pork Tenderloin	Garlic Butter Shrimp and Broccoli	Raspberry Coconut Chia Seed Pudding
11	Apple Cinnamon Quinoa Muffins	Zesty Baked Beef Thighs	Walnut-Crusted Baked Trout	Lemon Poppy Seed Muffins with Almond Flour
12	Smoked Salmon and Cream Cheese Bagel	Spaghetti Squash with Marinara Sauce	Rosemary Roasted Lamb Chops	Chocolate Avocado Pudding
13	Turkey and Vegetable Breakfast Skillet	Grilled Lemon Herb Pork Chops	Pistachio-Crusted Salmon	Strawberry and Almond Butter Bites
14	Veggie Breakfast Burrito with Whole Wheat Tortilla	Vegetable and Ground Beef Skillet	Sesame Ginger Glazed Tuna Steak	Greek Yogurt with Honey and Nuts
15	Whole Grain Toast with Smashed Avocado & Cherry Tomatoes	Cauliflower Fried Rice with Shrimp	Butternut Squash and Sage Risotto	Mango Sorbet with Lime Zest
16	Almond Butter & Banana Sandwich	Balsamic Glazed Pork Chops	Garlic and Herb Marinated Beef Kebabs	Avocado Chocolate Mousse
17	Quinoa Breakfast Porridge with Almonds	Garlic and Rosemary Roasted Pork Tenderloin	Spinach and Mushroom Stuffed Beef Rolls	Mixed Berry Sorbet
18	Sweet Potato Hash with Poached Eggs	Mushroom and Spinach Stuffed Pork Tenderloin	Coconut Lime Shrimp Stir-Fry	Chia Seed Pudding with Berries
19	Berry Smoothie Bowl with Chia Seeds	Barley and Mushroom Risotto	Grilled Lemon Herb Pork Chops	Dark Chocolate-Dipped Strawberries
20	Spinach and Feta Frittata	Herbed Grilled Pork Chops	Stuffed Bell Peppers with Lean Ground Beef	Berry Parfait with Greek Yogurt
21	Cucumber and Tomato Breakfast Salad	Whole Wheat Pasta with Tomato & Basil Sauce	Orange Glazed Grilled Swordfish	Almond Flour Blueberry Muffins

22	Cottage Cheese Pancakes with Berries	Teriyaki Glazed Tilapia	Citrus-Marinated Grilled Steak	Avocado Chocolate Mousse
23	Broccoli and Cheese Egg Muffins	Garlic Butter Shrimp and Broccoli	Lemon Rosemary Grilled Chicken Thighs	Raspberry Coconut Chia Seed Pudding
24	Avocado and Egg Breakfast Bowl	Beef and Vegetable Stir-Fry	Walnut-Crusted Baked Trout	Lemon Poppy Seed Muffins with Almond Flour
25	Apple Cinnamon Quinoa Muffins	Mediterranean Baked Salmon	Sesame Ginger Glazed Tuna Steak	Chocolate Avocado Pudding
26	Smoked Salmon and Cream Cheese Bagel	Spaghetti Squash with Marinara Sauce	Rosemary Roasted Lamb Chops	Strawberry and Almond Butter Bites
27	Turkey and Vegetable Breakfast Skillet	Grilled Lemon Herb Pork Chops	Pistachio-Crusted Salmon	Greek Yogurt with Honey and Nuts
28	Veggie Breakfast Burrito with Whole Wheat Tortilla	Vegetable and Ground Beef Skillet	Butternut Squash and Sage Risotto	Mango Sorbet with Lime Zest
29	Whole Grain Toast with Smashed Avocado & Cherry Tomatoes	Cauliflower Fried Rice with Shrimp	Garlic and Herb Marinated Beef Kebabs	Avocado Chocolate Mousse
30	Almond Butter & Banana Sandwich	Balsamic Glazed Pork Chops	Spinach and Mushroom Stuffed Beef Rolls	Mixed Berry Sorbet

Conversion Chart

Volume Equivalents (Liquid)

US Standard	US Standard (oz.)	Metric (approximate)
2 tbsps	1 fl. oz.	30 milliliter
¼ cup	2 fl. oz.	60 milliliter
½ cup	4 fl. oz.	120 milliliter
1 cup	8 fl. oz.	240 milliliter
1½ cups	12 fl. oz.	355 milliliter
2 cups or 1 pint	16 fl. oz.	475 milliliter
4 cups or 1 quart	32 fl. oz.	1 Liter
1 gallon	128 fl. oz.	4 Liter

Volume Equivalents (Dry)

US Standard	Metric (approximate)
⅛ tsp	0.5 milliliter
¼ tsp	1 milliliter
½ tsp	2 milliliter
¾ tsp	4 milliliter
1 tsp	5 milliliter
1 tbsp	15 milliliter
¼ cup	59 milliliter
⅓ cup	79 milliliter

½ cup	118 milliliter
⅔ cup	156 milliliter
¾ cup	177 milliliter
1 cup	235 milliliter
2 cups or 1 pint	475 milliliter
3 cups	700 milliliter
4 cups or 1 quart	1 Liter

Oven Temperatures

Fahrenheit (F)	Celsius (C) (approximate)
250 deg.F	120 deg.C
300 deg.F	150 deg.C
325 deg.F	165 deg.C
350 deg.F	180 deg.C
375 deg.F	190 deg.C
400 deg.F	200 deg.C
425 deg.F	220 deg.C
450 deg.F	230 deg.C

Weight Equivalents

US Standard	Metric (approximate)
1 tbsp	15 g
½ oz.	15 g
1 oz.	30 g
2 oz.	60 g
4 oz.	115 g
8 oz.	225 g
12 oz.	340 g
16 oz. or 1 lb.	455 g

DISCLAIMER:

Intended solely for the purpose of providing general information, the information contained in this book is presented here. It does not serve as a replacement for the diagnosis, treatment, or advice of a qualified medical practitioner. In the event that you have any inquiries concerning a medical problem, you should always consult with your primary care physician or another trained health expert. The author and publisher do not endorse specific diets, products, or treatments for diabetes, and individual results may vary. These are general guidelines based on the author's professional experience, and the recipes in this cookbook are recommendations for good cooking. It is important to seek the advice of a qualified medical practitioner prior to implementing any major alterations to your diet or lifestyle. This will ensure that the adjustments you make are suitable for your specific health requirements and circumstances. The author and publisher are not responsible for any adverse effect or consequences resulting from the use of the information presented in this book.

Made in the USA
Middletown, DE
22 May 2024

54708187R00068